5·13·14 Ingram $ 32.99

A Short Guide to a Long Life

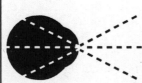

This Large Print Book carries the
Seal of Approval of N.A.V.H.

A SHORT GUIDE
TO A LONG LIFE

DAVID B. AGUS, MD
WITH KRISTIN LOBERG

Illustrations by Chieun Ko-Bistrong

THORNDIKE PRESS
A part of Gale, Cengage Learning

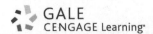

GALE
CENGAGE Learning·

Farmington Hills, Mich • San Francisco • New York • Waterville, Maine
Meriden, Conn • Mason, Ohio • Chicago

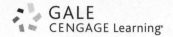
GALE
CENGAGE Learning®

LIBRARY OF CONGRESS CATALOGING-IN-PUBLICATION DATA

Agus, David, 1965– author.
    A short guide to a long life / by David B. Agus, MD with Kristin Loberg. — Large print edition.
        pages cm (Thorndike press large print health, home & learning)
    ISBN-13: 978-1-4104-6838-3 (hardcover)
    ISBN-10: 1-4104-6838-0 (hardcover)
    1. Longevity. 2. Aging—Nutritional aspects. 3. Physical fitness. 4. Self-care, Health. 5. Large type books. I. Loberg, Kristin, author. II. Title.
    RA776.75.A38 2014b
    613.2—dc23   2013050875

Published in 2014 by arrangement with Simon & Schuster, Inc.

Printed in the United States of America
1 2 3 4 5 6 7 18 17 16 15 14

To my wife, partner, and love,
Amy Povich,
and our genetic experiments gone right,
Sydney and Miles

A BRIEF HISTORICAL NOTE

Hippocrates was a Greek physician in the time of the third and fourth century BC. Modern medicine refers to Hippocrates as the father of Western medicine. He was among the first physicians to convey important "health rules" through his many now-famous quotes. Below are some examples that continue to have amazing relevance to today's medicine. In fact, one could argue that our modern world has brought science and data into the field, but his initial observations and recommendations were remarkably accurate over two thousand years ago.

Walking is man's best medicine.
Let food be thy medicine and medicine be
    thy food.
Declare the past, diagnose the present,
    foretell the future.
Primum non nocerum. (First, do no harm.)
It is far more important to know what

7

person the disease has than what disease the person has.

If we could give every individual the right amount of nourishment and exercise, not too little and not too much, we would have found the safest way to health.

A wise man should consider that health is the greatest of human blessings, and learn how by his own thought to derive benefit from his illnesses.

Everything in excess is opposed to nature.

To do nothing is also a good remedy.

There are in fact two things, science and opinion; the former begets knowledge, the latter ignorance.

Hippocrates (c. 460 BC–c. 370 BC)

CONTENTS

INTRODUCTION:
THE POWER OF PREVENTION

At least twice a week, I tell a patient that I have nothing left in my arsenal to combat his or her cancer. It's over, and in most cases the end is near. I've never gotten used to this gut-wrenching conversation. But I do it as part of the role I've accepted. That we are no better at treating cancer today, with a few notable exceptions, than we were fifty years ago is maddening. More infuriating still is that many of my patients could have prevented their cancer or other life-altering disease had they done a few things differently earlier in life. That makes those conversations even more upsetting. I'm pretty certain that most people could delay or totally prevent a vast majority of the illnesses we see today — including not only cancer but heart and kidney disease, stroke, obesity, diabetes, autoimmune disorders, and dementia and other neurodegenerative disorders — if they just adopt a few healthy habits early on and avoid the ones that lead to illness.

The best way to fight not just cancer but all the other ailments that typically develop over time is to prevent them. A staggering seven out of ten deaths among Americans each year are from chronic diseases like the ones I just named. Heart disease, cancer, and stroke account for more than 50 percent of all deaths every year. About half of us are living with a chronic condition right now.

But prevention is a hard sell. Think about yourself for a moment: can you see yourself twenty, thirty, or forty years from now? We all want to live however we choose today and pay our dues later. I see this payment being made by my patients daily, just by looking into their eyes.

I'd like nothing more than to be put out of my job. Imagine a world where we all die of old age — our bodies go kaput, much like an old car with hundreds of thousands of great miles on it. One day, the engine doesn't start and nothing can revive it. In fact, 1951 was the last year you could die in the United States with the cause "old age" being listed on the death certificate. Since then, we've had to name a specific disease, injury, or complication. I find it astonishing to think that we live in a high-tech world with access to a vast array of knowledge about how to stay healthy, and yet preventable noncommunicable diseases now account for more deaths worldwide than all other causes combined. We rarely hear about the person who dies peacefully in her sleep at ninety-nine years young. Instead, we hear about individuals who suffer mightily and eventually succumb after a long "battle."

In our age of information, where health tips are dispensed like candy by the media, the work of being healthy has gotten complicated. Just consider your own search for truth about what's good for you — or what's bad. It's common practice to rely on experts to tell us how to live — news stories covering the latest scientific findings, bestselling books that tout one theory or another, government recommendations, claims on labels, and doctors like me. But this advice is so terribly common that it commonly conflicts. What is a person to do with a hot media account of a new study that finds multivitamins effective in preventing cancer — only to read another media account the next day that says multivitamins can increase your risk for cancer and do nothing for heart health? (And to add insult to injury, you learn that the company that makes the vitamins is the same one that makes the drugs to combat cancer!)

When I wrote my first book, *The End of Illness,* my purpose was simple: to share what I'd learned from working out on the edge of the cliff that is the war on cancer — a place where we take risks in medicine in the hope of finding innovations to prolong people's lives. While the death rate from cancer hasn't changed dramatically in the past fifty years, progress against other diseases has relied on single discoveries that have allowed us to treat or eradicate them. Examples include the use of statins to prevent cardiovascular disease and stroke, antibiotics to combat infectious diseases originating from bacteria, antivirals and vaccines to tackle and protect against specific viruses, and a heightened awareness of the risks posed by behavioral factors such as smoking and poor diet or overeating. Except for these isolated improvements, why aren't we better at treating and curing chronic degenerative diseases that often cannot be blamed on a single culprit?

For decades we've tried to reduce our understanding of the body and its potential breakdowns to a finite cause, be it a mutation, a germ, a deficiency, or a number such as a white blood cell count, glucose level, or a triglyceride value. But this has led us far astray from a perspective that could not only change how we care for the body, but also how we create the next generation of treatments and, in some instances, cures. The original title of *The End of Illness,* upon which this life guide is based, was *What Is Health?* It's a question that bugs me and my colleagues to this day. I don't know what true health is. We can certainly try to measure health in a variety of ways — weight, cholesterol, blood sugar, blood cell count, how you look, and how well you sleep, for example. But that doesn't really tell me much in terms of overall health and how many years and days you might have left. This has motivated me to urge people to begin viewing their total health as a complex network of processes that cannot be explained by looking at any one pathway or focal point. In many instances, it does no good to try to understand a certain disease; we just need to control it, much like an air traffic controller manages planes without knowing exactly how to fly one. This radically different perspective on health is what can open the doorway to future solutions, and even cures.

I don't think I fully grasped the thorniness surrounding the subject of health, however, until I started discussing my book and responding to readers. I quickly found myself on the receiving end of questions like, What's your real motivation for writing a book? Why are you hawking prescription drugs? How can a doctor who treats the very rich have anything valuable to give the average person who barely has health insurance? Let me head this last question off at the pass right now by saying the vast majority of my "prescriptions" in this book are surprisingly simple, such as wearing good shoes (Rule 59) and eating lunch at the same time every day (Rule 3). How much does it cost to keep a fairly regular schedule every day and to walk around more (Rule 16)? Put another way, how much will you save by ditching your vitamins and supplements (Rule 62)? How much easier will your life get once you learn that it's better to buy frozen vegetables than some fresh produce (which isn't nearly as fresh as you think; see Rule 5). And even when I suggest something that comes with a price, such as paying for a DNA screening test, there's often an inexpensive, if not totally free, alternative (see Rule 19), which can be even more informative and useful.

When I went on the *Dr. Oz Show* in the fall of 2012, I was billed as the most controversial doctor in America. But I think I'm the absolute opposite. I won't endorse anything that's not backed by well-controlled clinical trials — studies that live up to the rigors of the scientific method. In that regard, I'm one of the most conservative of doctors in America. People tend to label certain things as aggressive or, conversely, mainstream. Many individuals think taking aspirin and statins on a daily basis is aggressive but taking vitamins is mainstream. But the data tell a totally different story, painting a picture in which aspirin and statins can significantly *reduce* your risk of death (what scientists call "all cause mortality") while vitamins and supplements may *raise* your risk for a variety of illnesses, including cancer. I can understand and appreciate someone's suspicion when hearing a doctor push a pill, and her assumption that there must be financial remuneration or incentive involved. For the record, I have no financial ties to any drug company. In the past I have been paid for giving lectures to pharmaceutical management teams, but I've never been involved with any pharmaceutical marketing. If I suggest a certain drug or class of drugs, it's for a good, well-documented reason: because they have been shown to make a positive difference.

I actually don't mind stirring up controversy and inspiring people to ask questions. Spending on food and health together make up more than 30 percent of the U.S. economy, yet our politicians and civic leaders aren't discussing these important issues. They may bicker about how to finance health-care reform, but I'd like to see more attention on the reform itself. It boggles my mind to think the conversation remains stuck on figuring out how to pay for health care rather than on diminishing our need for it. Indeed, part of my motivation in writing this book is to make you — the health-care consumer — an agent of change, starting with yourself. Each one of us can make a difference if we each are part of reducing the overall demand for health care. The result will follow one of the fundamental laws of Econ 101: when we start living strong, robust lives, we'll lessen our need for health care, causing the demand to decrease and costs to go down. Simple as that.

The other chief reason for writing this book is probably pretty obvious: I want these rules to reach as many people as possible. After *The End of Illness* came out, many people asked me to distill my Health Rules down to a prescriptive list for them to keep on hand. They wanted a cheat sheet. In my previous book, I spent a lot of time going through the evidence; I won't be doing that here. I also won't be using any medical terminology or fancy language to convey my ideas. This is as pure and direct as it gets — less about theory, research, history, and science and more about the basic practices you can follow in your daily life. Nothing is meant to be a rigid directive. Of all the rules I present, the most important one is this: you have to find what works for you. The sixty-five rules here are each accompanied by a paragraph or two of explanation. A few, however, require little or no clarification (Rule 29: Smile) and I hope you just accept them at face value.

My goal is that this book will allow you to take the confusion out of knowing how to live to be healthy — to feel as fabulous as possible at any age. As I said in my previous book:

My recommendations won't be terribly exacting. I'm not interested in telling you how to live your life or what you should be eating for dinner. I'm also not here to diagnose you. Instead, I want to empower you to take control over your body and the future of your health. The suggestions offered here are more like lifestyle algorithms — mental devices for thinking through our myriad lifestyle choices. Those choices must be tempered by our values and individual codes of ethics and behavior. Because there is no single answer to the question of what is health, these guidelines will produce as many different "healthy styles" as there are people living them.

My objective is to help you make the most of your health, whether or not you're currently battling an illness. I'd like to encourage you to take a hard look at your understanding of health and open up your mind to a change in perspective. It can significantly improve your life.

That we need simple reminders of what it means to live a healthy life despite the volume of advice transmitted daily in the media is a telling sign of our confusion. I can only hope that as you read this book you gain not only the knowledge you need to take advantage of modern science and medicine, but also the wisdom to discern the good from the questionable to make the best decisions for yourself. I also hope that your future will be determined by the power of choice, and, when necessary, that it will guide you down pathways of healing. Only you can end illness.

I've divided this book into three sections. The first, "What to Do," gives a clear set of just that — things you can do that will make you the architect of your health kingdom. The second part, "What to Avoid," offers my rules for the things to stay away from that can harm your health. Some of these will be obvious, such as limiting risky behaviors and avoiding less-than-perfect ingredients in foods, but some won't be so apparent, such as how not to fall prey to hyperbole in the media and how not to hoard your medical information. I'm going to help you learn how to separate the hype from the helpful and see the ways in which you can benefit from sharing your medical information with the world. Part three, "Doctor's Orders," makes my recommendations even more straightforward by listing out a plan based on which decade you're in (twenties, thirties, forties, and so on). This is your real cheat sheet — the bulleted list of agenda items you should tend to at each particular age. The nature of this book's structure and content makes for some repeated ideas, and two different rules may take you to the same place. My hope is that presenting these principles in different ways will make them more memorable. Enjoy the read, and I trust that a handful of these rules will stick with you and improve your life.

Before we begin, let me first present important ground rules.

Ground Rule 1

Health information is a moving target. Recommendations today may change tomorrow. For now, the following rules are relevant based on the data we have available that convincingly show the best practices for reducing your risk of disease. While it's true that you can find single, unrepeated studies that contradict my ideas, that's not how science works. When scientists weigh in on a topic, they can't just rely on single studies that support their view. Instead, they have to consider all the studies on a topic and examine the results of each. That is exactly what a meta-analysis does. Hence, all of my prescriptions are rooted in studies that meet this gold standard. They always will be. And if the day comes when science uproots an established "truth" or does a complete 180 on a universally accepted fact, then I will welcome that new viewpoint with excitement and resolve (and a new rule).

Ground Rule 2

The rules in this book are not meant to be blanket recommendations, especially when it comes to prescription medications. The point is to have a discussion about them with your doctor and family, and also to consider your inner core values. So take the time to sit, think, and talk through any new direction you decide to take in your life. Remember, too, that health is in constant flux (see Ground Rule 1). You need to adapt to changes as you age. In science-speak we say that humans are "emergent systems" — they are constantly changing, developing, and evolving. The body is an incredible self-regulating machine. You don't need to do much to support its health and optimal wellness. In the last hour, for instance, about one billion cells were replaced in your body without your having to think about it.

Ground Rule 3

You are in charge of you. This book is designed as a manual to help you know when to be introspective and when to question things. If I suggest something that offends you or that you flatly reject, just move on. At the heart of my message is the importance of knowing how to have a productive conversation with yourself and your physician; it's also about raising your awareness about the things you do today that affect your tomorrows. When you come across a rule that makes you feel uncomfortable, remember that none of these is absolutely perfect. Instead of dismissing it, ask for better studies and, in turn, better technology. We have to be pushing for progress. Here's a quick example: aspirin may be touted as a miracle drug (Rule 22), but it's still flawed, given the side effects it can cause, namely bleeding and upset stomach. We should question why the National Institutes of Health doesn't spend large sums on making better aspirin so we can reap its miraculous benefits minus the potential side effects.

One final confession: I admit that I was so moved by Michael Pollan's *Food Rules,* which was inspired by his bestselling *In Defense of Food: An Eater's Manifesto,* that his book provided the model for this one. I reference Pollan a few times in *The End of Illness,* for I deeply respect his take on dietary issues and think he states the facts brilliantly. So as much as *Food Rules* lays out a set of concise, memorable rules for eating wisely, my *Short Guide to a Long Life* similarly presents my set of rules for *living* wisely. This of course will include a few rules about eating and buying food, but I will also address all the other factors that play into good health. I've done my best to keep it short and sweet, while still keeping my promise to bestow on you the recipe for a long and healthy life.

■ ■ ■ ■

PART I
WHAT TO DO

■ ■ ■ ■

1
Listen, Look, Feel
(and Record Your
Body's Features)

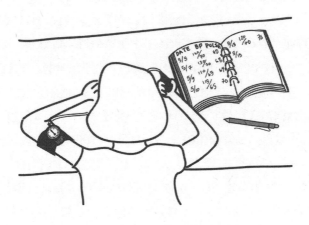

These days it's easier to know your blood pressure and heart rate than it is to find a pay phone. If I had to put one rule above all others, it would be this: get to know yourself. It's why I'm starting this entire list of things to do with a directive to take inventory of your body's features, character-istics, vital signs, and other health param-eters that are relatively easy to obtain. Let's bring the concept of *listen, look, and feel* home. Obviously, aim for the measurements you can take with tools at your fingertips or at a local pharmacy, or that don't require any hardware at all, just your inner thoughts and sensations. Include notes such as how you feel in general, how well you're sleeping, whether you harbor any aches and pains, and what kinds of activities or foods seem to irritate your body. How many of us never stop and ask: Do I feel healthy? Is it hard for me to get out of bed in the morning? Is there a pattern to the times when I feel lousy and, conversely, fantastic? You'd be surprised by how effortless it can be to decode the mysteries of your own body's quirks and rhythms just by tuning in!

If you want to get more technical, then gather clues to your body's signals by recording the following information daily over the course of three months: the time of day, your blood pressure, your pulse, and what's going on at that time (e.g., you just ate breakfast, you're anxious upon waking up, you're relaxed in front of the television, or you've received a piece of bad news in the mail). Pick different times of the day to do your self-examination, as this will inform you of times when, say, your blood pressure is high or your mood is low. You'll then want to repeat this exercise throughout the year, preferably once every couple of months, to note changes. Don't wait until you're in the doctor's office, which is typically a rare occasion for most of us. Do, however, bring your personal health diary with you to share at your next appointment. You can buy or access equipment to take your blood pressure at most pharmacies, and some tools can even be downloaded as an application for your smart phone (see Rule 2).

I'm a big believer in what's called personalized medicine, which means customizing your health care to your specific needs based on your physiology, genetics, value system, and individual circumstances. Medicine is finally at a place where we have the technology to tailor treatment and preventive protocols to an individual, just like a seamstress can tailor a garment to a person's body. But it all begins with you. You won't be able to enjoy the benefits of personalized medicine until you take a close look at your unique body.

Below is a list of general questions to ask yourself during your personal checkup every couple of months after you've completed the intense three-month initiation diary: [*]

---

[*] Go to www.davidagus.com for a free comprehensive, downloadable questionnaire.

- How would you rank your overall energy levels?
- Anything abnormal to report (skin, hair, sensations, breathing, appetite, digestion)?
- Do you suffer from any chronic conditions?
- How bad is your stress level on a scale of 1 to 10?
- Are you happy?
- What do you want to change in your life?
- What is your weight? (Aim to measure your weight once a week or every two weeks.)

Of course, these questions should also be asked on day 1. And be honest.

2
MEASURE YOURSELF

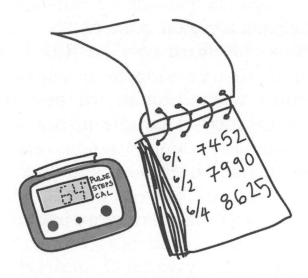

Every day I read about some new gadget or app on the market that can help track my health and happiness. (At last count, there were more than seven thousand self-tracking smart-phone apps alone, and the market for self-tracking gadgetry is exploding.)

How many steps did you take today? How long were you in dreamy REM sleep last night? How fast did you eat lunch? What's your pulse? How many calories are you burning? What's your blood oxygen level? What's your brain's electrical activity at night? How stressed are you? What emotions are you feeling? You can answer these questions if you have the right device. (Although I should hope you can take a good guess as to how stressed and emotional you are sans a digital reader.)

If you really want to take Rule 1 to the maximum, then consider measuring yourself a bit more formally with the help of nifty devices. In 2007, a couple of brainy *Wired* editors saw this coming: the day when we'd be able to track ourselves digitally as Sanctorius of Padua did manually when he weighed everything that came in and out of his body over a period of thirty years in the sixteenth and seventeenth centuries. The *Wired* editors coined the term the "quantified self," and this kind of effort has already become a movement. Even if you don't subscribe to the idea of wearing a piece of Star Treky equipment, most of us keep mental track of certain things in our lives such as weight, sleep quality, and activity level — if just to make sure we're within the parameters we'd like to follow.

But seriously, you might want to consider

adding a tracking app or device of some kind to your life. I can't even begin to list them all here, and by the time you read this a whole new generation of useful software programs and devices will surely have hit the market. You can track, calculate, plan, and research just about anything health related these days and personalize that info. Some apps can be programmed for your location and, say, notify you of the foods in your geographical area that are in season and provide information on local farmers markets. Pretty soon we'll be able to wear little devices that can clue us in to our body's dynamics all day long. Not that we all may want to wear such gadgets 24/7, but these could be incredibly powerful tools for creating and maintaining baseline numbers, and in some cases for training ourselves to know when we could benefit from some behavioral modifications. It's hard to take yourself from a raging bull in terms of stress back down to a calm, cool cucumber, but if a device or app could alert you that you're entering a danger zone, it might motivate you to make effective changes to reduce your stress.

Tools are critical to our success in so many areas in life — e-mail and cell phones allow us to communicate, the Internet to research, cars to get where we are going. Why would we think that we don't need such help with our health? The tools are already at our disposal. They aren't meant to make us totally self-absorbed; they are meant to help us take better care of ourselves. Using them will propagate the incentives we need. Make it a goal to study yourself consistently and keep charts. Listen to your body, and remember — only you know your body best.

For a constantly updated list of interesting apps and devices, go to http://davidagus .com/mhealth.

3
AUTOMATE YOUR LIFE

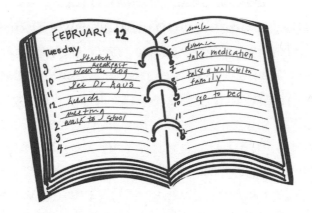

Your body loves predictability. Did you get up today at the same time as yesterday? Will you eat your next meal at roughly the same time you ate that meal yesterday? One of the best ways of reducing stress on your body and keeping its preferred, balanced state of being (homeostasis) is to maintain a regular, consistent routine on a daily basis, 365 days a year, to the best of your ability. Yes, regardless of weekends, holidays, social demands, late nights at the office, and other body-busting, schedule-disrupting events.

The four chief areas where you can make great strides in honoring your body's homeostasis are your sleep-wake cycles, eating times, periods of physical activity, and schedule for taking any prescribed medications. Just as your body aches for a consistent sleep schedule, it also craves a regular eating routine. If you were to step into a body that's been deprived of its expectation of eating lunch at noon, for example, you'd witness biological activities going on that would likely surprise you. Your body won't just show signs of hunger; it will also experience a surge in cortisol, the stress hormone that tells your body to hold tightly to fat and to conserve energy. In other words, if you don't eat when your body anticipates food, it will sabotage your efforts to lose or maintain an ideal weight.

By the same token, don't throw a wrench into that finely tuned body of yours by sporadic snacking or eating randomly when you're not hungry just to counteract an emotional state such as boredom, loneliness, or depression. If you don't normally snack at 3:00 p.m. every single day, then don't reach for that apple fritter to lift your late-afternoon lull. But if you need an afternoon snack, have it at a regular time. And go for a handful of nuts, a piece of whole fruit, veggies dipped in hummus, or some cheese and crackers rather than the processed fried dough.

4
MOBILIZE YOUR MEDICAL DATA

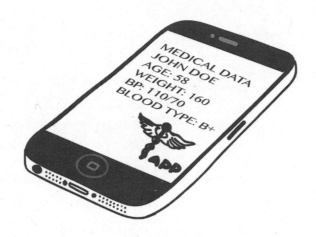

Do you have copies of all your medical records, and are they accessible online somewhere? Why not? What if you land in the emergency room and cannot talk but have a potentially fatal allergy to penicillin — the very drug a doctor is about to inject into you?

We use our phones and computers today for just about everything, with one exception: storing our medical records and keeping our health information updated. Aim to have all your records stored in your "mobile cloud" so they are always accessible to you. Give a trusted family member (spouse, parent, sibling, adult child) or friend your passwords so they can access those same files when and if it becomes necessary. Everyone needs a partner in health care. Pick someone. Give that person full access to all of the places where you keep your medical data. If you don't have your medical records nicely organized in digital files, request copies of your files from your doctors. Spend a weekend afternoon creating digital copies of them using a scanner. You can also keep them on a USB key chain that you take everywhere. This task may sound daunting, but it's just a few hours of work from which you can benefit for the rest of your life. It is unusual that patients of mine have a medical emergency between the hours of 9:00 a.m. and 5:00 p.m. when the office is open and we can access their records. Problems always seem to happen in the middle of the night, on a weekend, or when someone is traveling! We each have different health profiles, but that distinctiveness can present a challenge to doctors who don't know anything about us, yet have been given the job of treating us. Having your entire medical record on file to hand over just might save your life.

5

EAT REAL FOOD (AND DON'T LET THE APPLE FALL FAR FROM THE TREE)

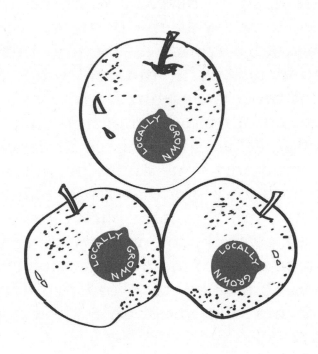

The best way to summarize the sad need for this rule is simply to quote Michael Pollan from his book *In Defense of Food:* "That anyone should need to write a book advising people to 'eat food' could be taken as a measure of our alienation and confusion."

And indeed, every day people ask the question, What should I eat?

Answer: real food.

What constitutes real food? With the exception of flash-frozen fruits and vegetables, anything that *doesn't* come with a label or an FDA-approved nutrition facts label is likely to be real, as ironic as that sounds. If you walk the perimeter of your grocery store (produce section, butcher, fishmonger), you'll find real food. Steer clear of those aisles lined with boxes and bottles and other food impostors that come in pretty packages. If you read a label that lists ingredients you cannot pronounce or define without a graduate-level textbook in chemistry, put that item back on the shelf and walk away! Focus on consuming foods that are as close to nature as possible, which will also help you to avoid problematic ingredients that you don't know you're sensitive to.

Watch out for health claims, too. If a food product has to tell you that it's good for you (with descriptions and health claims on their packaging that say things like "low fat!" "low in sugar!" "lite," "cholesterol free!" "baked not fried," "antioxidant rich," and "all natural"), then it's probably not very real. Think about it: in order for claims to be made, the food must be packaged somehow and pass some sort of test or criteria for the seal of approval. This means that the food cannot possibly be all that real and as close to nature as possible. Orange juice, for instance, will come with lots of health claims ("a full day's worth of vitamin C!"), but the quiet, lonely whole orange sitting in a produce basket will do more for your health than an eight-ounce glass of fiberless fructose. If they have to tell you why you should be eating it, you *shouldn't* be eating it. What's more, many people think they are eating healthily when they buy diet frozen dinners, fat-free ice cream or frozen yogurt, 100 percent natural fruit juice, low-fat cheese, energy bars, diet soda, organic hundred-calorie snack packs, and so on. But if you look at the nutritional content of these foods, and the order in which the ingredients are listed, which reflects their prevalence, you're likely to find more sugar, saturated fat, salt, and ingredients with weird names than anything else.

And one more note about this rule: go for seasonal items when you buy fresh produce. If you find yourself eating blueberries and heirloom tomatoes in February or brussels sprouts and kiwifruit in June, then you're likely eating fruits and veggies that have fallen too far from the tree. In other words, they have traveled a long way to get to your GPS coordinates. The minute a fruit or vegetable is picked is the moment it starts to change chemically and lose nutritional value. Too many fruits and vegetables are available year-round now thanks to shipping technologies. We may live in a world where we can access pretty much any type of food all year long, but it comes at a major expense: nutrition. By the time the vast majority of produce reaches the bins and aisles of your local supermarket, it doesn't contain nearly the same amount of nutrients as when plucked from the plant or yanked from its roots. If fruits and vegetables are picked before they are ripe — which many of them are to help them endure the long shipment — they have less time to develop a full spectrum of vitamins and minerals. The produce might look ripe on the outside, but it will never have the same nutritive value as it would have if it had been allowed to ripen fully before harvest. In addition, during the long haul from farm to fork, fresh fruits and vegetables are exposed to lots of heat and light, which also degrade some nutrients, especially delicate vitamins such as C and the B vitamin thiamine. What we end up with in our mouths is a nutrient-poor product that may also contain some chemicals that we would like to avoid.

Unless you can buy truly fresh produce that's in season and has been delivered recently from a nearby farm, head on over to your grocer's freezer section and opt for frozen fruits and vegetables, often labeled as "fresh flash-frozen." Fruits and vegetables chosen for freezing tend to be plucked or picked at their peak ripeness, a time when — as a general rule — they are packed with the most nutrients. Eat fruits and vegetables soon after purchase, including the frozen variety. Over many months, even the nutrients in frozen vegetables inevitably degrade. And for produce that you can buy truly fresh, please don't insult the sweet fruit and vibrant veggies by letting them languish in your kitchen's fruit bowl or crisper in the refrigerator. Enjoy them as soon as possible.

All of this leads us to the question, How can you know what's truly fresh? Ah, see the next rule.

6
KNOW YOUR GROCER

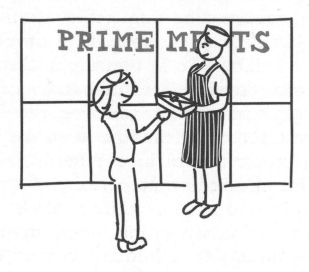

Short of being a farmer who knows exactly what's in season, you can learn all the information you need to make smart purchases just by chatting up your local grocer. The people who stock the produce section, for instance, will tell you what just came in, where it came from, and how it was farmed. The guy manning the butcher counter can share details about the ranchers who supplied the meat, and the woman behind the fish counter can offer information as to which fish is the freshest, most sustainably caught. Don't be intimidated by these folks. They love imparting their knowledge.

And when you do venture out of the grocery store and into your local farmers market, that's where you'll want to introduce yourself to the people who are that much closer to the source of your food. Get to know your local farmers as you would your grocer. Farmers markets rarely sell imported items, so what you find there will be the freshest possible. If you can buy most of your fresh produce from a local farmers market, you can automatically avoid the nutrient-poor, processed, nonseasonal fare. You may have to spend a little more for your groceries, but this is when it really counts. You get what you pay for: you'll be eating high-quality foods and enjoying a high quality of life that won't cost you bundles in health-care bills for illnesses you could have avoided. Besides, high-quality food just tastes better, so you're more likely to be satisfied with less of it, thereby controlling your calories.

7
GROW A GARDEN

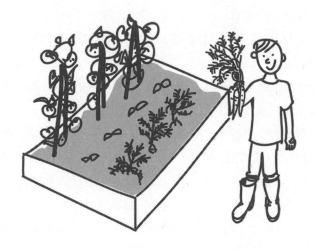

This should be a mandatory rule for anyone with children, especially young ones. I know of no better way to teach principles of health and good eating than to show kids what real food looks like in the growing phase. This will force you to learn what blooms in May versus what crops up in December. And there's just nothing you can buy in the grocery store or even at your farmers market that compares nutritionwise with food you pick a few feet from your kitchen and use immediately for cooking or just eat raw.

Don't panic if you live in an itty-bitty apartment or lack a green thumb. Be willing to experiment and start with easy plants that work in your climate and space. Your local nursery will be able to give you all the details and equipment you need (think pots, soil, seeds). You needn't own an acre or have a huge amount of unused area in your yard. A simple window box will suffice. And you can just start by growing herbs and spices (parsley, basil, mint, sage), then graduate to some of the more advanced crops as your space allows, such as peppers, tomatoes, cucumbers, green beans, snow peas, lettuce, and Swiss chard. In some places, you can grow a garden all year round and rotate which crops you're cultivating based on the season. Better yet, make this a community effort and join forces with neighbors. Split up who grows what and share in the bounty. Now, that's neighborly for a good cause: community health.

8
MAINTAIN A DIETARY PROTOCOL THAT WORKS FOR YOU

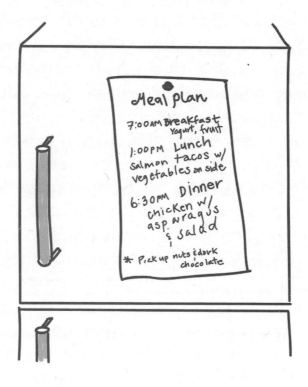

Should you eat gluten free? Low carb? Vegan? Raw? Low fat? Follow Weight Watchers? In truth, it doesn't really matter as long as you enjoy what you're eating, your body seems to love it, and you're not forcing yourself to adhere to an impossibly strict protocol that probably lacks certain nutrients by virtue of its restrictions. Just as there are many religions in the world, there are many healthy eating traditions, and it is worth remembering why they have worked through the centuries.

I love how Michael Pollan puts it in his forty-eighth food rule: "Eat More Like the French. Or the Japanese. Or the Italians. Or the Greeks." Any traditional diet will beat out our processed food culture, and traditional eating habits have worked for centuries among different peoples (with vastly different diets) around the world. These habits include moderating portions, sharing food at a communal table, not going back for seconds, and letting hunger build up in between meals (no snacking). Today, a great part of our larger-than-life waistlines is due not only to poor dietary choices but also to poor eating habits. We eat in solitude on the go, in our cars, and at our desks. Seldom do we sit around the table and linger over lively conversations with loved ones. And we go back for second and third (and fourth) helpings as if the food is unlimited (because it pretty much is). We also avoid the sensation of hunger by eating randomly throughout the day, mindlessly downing lots of snacks. Or, on the other end of the spectrum, if we skip meals and save our caloric load for a banquet at night, we're more likely to overindulge and then have trouble sleeping. So always leave the dinner table a little hungry (and leave something on your plate — a clean plate is not always a happy plate!).

One of the easiest ways to gain control of the ideal diet for you is simply to cook more. Make your own food. Enjoy it with others at a table (not a desk, in front of the television, or behind the wheel). Borrow recipes from around the world and buy fresh ingredients. I'll even give you permission to eat as many snack foods and delectable desserts as you like so long as you make them from scratch using real ingredients and have them at a daily regular snack time. Then abide by the same portion control rules you'd use for any regular meal, treating treats as treats, and you'll have accomplished more than the vast majority of Americans.

9
CULTIVATE OM IN THE OFFICE

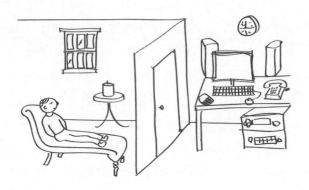

It shouldn't take a study to highlight the negative impact work-related stress can have on us physically, but now we can point to several, one of which was done recently in Finland that showed just how bad job stress can be. In 2012, Finnish researchers examined nearly three thousand people and correlated stress on the job with faster biological aging. How exactly did they calculate this? They measured these people's telomeres — DNA sequences found at the end of a person's chromosomes and whose lengths can be associated with aging, risk of illness, and possibly death. The theory put simply is that the shorter your telomeres, the shorter your life. And it turns out that the more pressure you feel at work, the more likely that your telomeres will shorten. In addition to this correlative relationship on your telomeres, there is the increased risk for heart trouble when you carry so much stress. It's practically cliché now to say that stress causes heart disease, but it's true. The heart may be among the strongest, most invincible organs in our body — after all, it pumps about 2,000 gallons of blood each day and beats, on average, more than 100,000 times daily — but that doesn't mean it's immune to things as subtle as psychological stress. It's no surprise that we're most likely to suffer a heart attack on a Monday, the first day of the workweek.

Job strain is a part of life. So what can we do to ease the pressure? Maintain simple routines at work that lift your mood and keep things in perspective. Some ideas: go for a walk during lunch in the bright sun; walk around more in the office and take your calls while standing up and moving around; take a deep breath before answering the phone; play relaxing music while working; skip happy hour and go to the gym to burn off steam instead; take scheduled time-outs during the day when you visit your favorite blogger or website for a few minutes; and decide when you check e-mail and respond to messages. The average working professional spends roughly 23 percent of the workday on e-mail and glances at the inbox about thirty-six times an hour. It takes most of us more than a minute to return to a task once we've stopped to read a new e-mail. And that can add stress.

10
HAVE A GLASS OF
WINE WITH DINNER

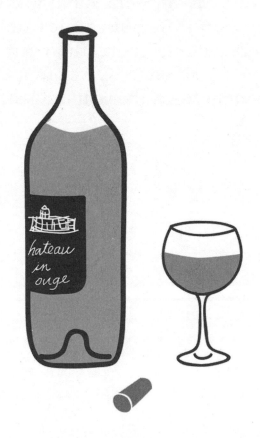

Habits that transcend culture and religion and date back thousands of years probably have some benefit to them regardless of what the science says. But now we know that moderate alcohol intake, especially from red wine, can reduce one's risk for heart disease. This benefit does have a caveat, however: drinking can potentially increase one's risk for breast cancer, and drinking too much is far worse for your heart than being a teetotaler. How do you find the sweet spot? Aim for no more than one drink a day if you're a woman and two if you're a man. And if you abstain during the workweek, you don't have permission to binge drink over the weekend.

11
PRACTICE GOOD HYGIENE — IN BED AND OUT

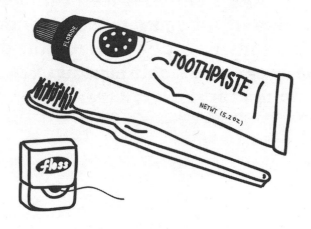

Good health starts with good hygiene. It's hard to believe that the dramatic decrease in infectious diseases between the discovery of germs and antidotes such as antibiotics and vaccines was actually not the result of high-tech medical treatments, but rather of changes in how we practice good hygiene. Although technically not a discovery on par with penicillin and the smallpox or polio vaccines, the mid-nineteenth-century recognition of the importance of hand washing was a huge medical breakthrough that saved a lot of people long before vaccines and antibiotics were widely available.

In 1847, while working at an obstetrics clinic in Vienna, Hungarian-born physician Dr. Ignaz Semmelweis noticed that fatal fevers among mothers of newborn children happened more frequently in birthings assisted by medical students than in those assisted by midwives. This prompted him to look closer at the clinic's practices, and he soon noted that the medical students who aided in childbirth often did so after performing autopsies on people who had died from bacterial sepsis — a whole-body blood infection in which the inflammatory response to a blooming bacteria turns deadly. He then established a strict policy of hand washing with a chlorinated antiseptic solution, and lo and behold, mortality rates dropped ten- to twentyfold within three months. It was proof that the transfer of disease could be significantly reduced by this simple hygienic practice, even though doctors at the time didn't know the exact causes of such diseases in many cases. Had civilization figured this out sooner, perhaps we could have avoided many of the deaths associated with plagues and epidemics that wiped out millions of people in earlier centuries.

Even today, we are inclined to trivialize the simple act of hand washing and would do well to keep it at the top of our priorities on a daily basis. You'll give yourself an advantage in avoiding germs that can make you sick, and you'll help prevent the spread of germs to others. All you need is a dollop of soap and water. Antimicrobial soaps aren't necessary; the standard stuff is just as good. But if you don't have access to water, then use an alcohol-based hand sanitizer. Some studies have shown that people who washed their hands at least five times a day were 35 percent less likely to catch the flu than those who lathered up less.

In addition to hand hygiene, maintaining general hygiene throughout your body will go a long way to protect you from the ick factor — think about head lice, bad breath, body odor, pinworms, and athlete's foot. All of these can largely be controlled just by practicing good hygiene. Don't forget to tend to cuts and scrapes immediately with antiseptics and bandages, no matter how trivial they seem. This will help you to avoid dangerous skin infections such as a painful staph invasion from hard-to-kill bacteria that can require serious oral antibiotics later on. And what about bed hygiene? Restful sleep starts with a clean and tidy bedroom. Wash your sheets in hot water once a week and keep clutter and electronics out. This habit will help you to practice good sleep hygiene (see Rule 58).

12
COHABITATE

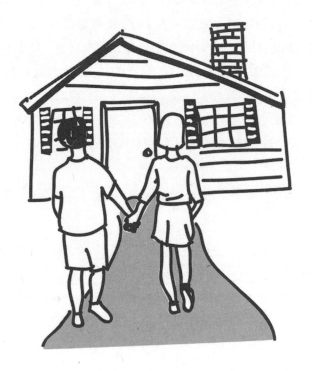

While at first blush it may seem unlikely that a connection has been found between cohabitation and longevity, consider the following: when you live with someone else, you have a reason to pay more attention to your health and hygiene. You've got another person to hold you accountable for your actions and lifestyle habits. You're less likely to engage in risky behaviors. And you're more likely to have a built-in system for coping with stress, because another warm human body is present in your daily life. If you come home mad, frustrated, and on the verge of a breakdown, you've at least got a sounding board. Which might explain why happy cohabitating couples repeatedly score better on blood pressure tests than their single counterparts. Whether or not this rule should entail marriage is up to you. And whether it should include children is another thing to consider (see Rule 47).

13
Maintain a Healthy Weight

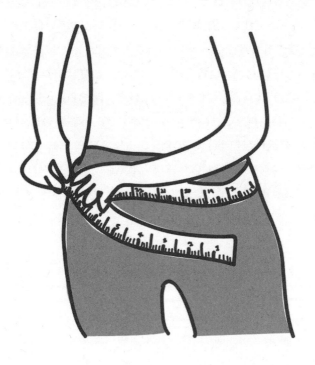

It should come as no surprise that a healthy weight corresponds to a healthy body. When the body is saddled with too many pounds (or, on the other end of the spectrum, too few pounds), it cannot function optimally.

Here's another way to look at it: each pound of weight lost equals a four-pound reduction in the knee load for every step you take. So if you take ten thousand steps a day, that translates to a twenty-ton reduction in the pressure on your knees. Think of that cumulative effect over a whole year! Even a small weight loss makes a big difference in the long run.

Being overweight increases your risk for virtually all illnesses and chronic conditions, from the obvious ones like heart disease, arthritis, and diabetes to dementia and cancer. Don't know if you're at a healthy weight? Search for a body mass index (BMI) calculator and chart online and see how you match up. The goal is to maintain a BMI of between 18.5 and 24.9. The National Heart, Lung and Blood Institute has a good one at http://nhlbisupport.com/bmi.

14
GET YOUR ANNUAL FLU SHOT, EVEN IF YOU "NEVER GET SICK" AND "HAVE NEVER GOTTEN THE FLU"

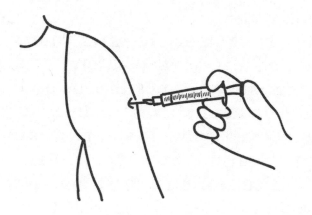

If you could take an inexpensive pill once a year that would help prevent all forms of cancer and has zero side effects, you'd probably consider it. Well, that's what a flu shot has the potential to do. It's a simple annual vaccine that will go a long way in protecting you from getting terribly sick for days, if not weeks, during which you cannot work, focus, fulfill your household duties, hang out with family members and friends, and enjoy life as usual. But immunizing yourself against influenza isn't just about beating the flu. A mere one to two weeks of an inflammatory storm, which is what will take place in your body if you contract the flu, can harm you in ways that increase your lifetime risk for obesity and many illnesses, including heart attack, strokes, and cancer.

For years now the American Heart Association and the American College of Cardiology have recommended flu vaccines for anyone with heart disease because it's been shown to prevent fatal heart attacks and strokes and even reduce the risk of death from any illness. In 2012, a study emerged showing that pregnant women who suffer through the flu have a significantly increased risk of having a child with autism. So imagine what the vaccine can do for a healthy individual hoping to avoid all these ills. (An idea: since we know the flu shot can lessen the risk for obesity, perhaps we should campaign for it by saying it will keep you thin! How many people would show up at the immunization clinic?) Sadly, people still cling to false notions that the flu vaccine has side effects, that it doesn't work, that it can *cause* the flu, or that it contains toxins or poisons. Malarkey. Most disturbing of all is that the people who seem to harbor these irrational notions are often the most educated. To say "I never get a flu shot and I never get the flu" is like declaring "I eat cheeseburgers and fries every day, don't exercise, and I've never gotten fat or had a heart attack."

There is nothing heroic about resisting the flu shot and then powering through the flu if you contract it. Influenza kills as many as forty-five thousand Americans a year, and the vaccine reduces deaths, illnesses, the use of antibiotics, and the number of hospital visits. Getting the shot isn't just about you; it can greatly lessen the burdens on our health-care system and can protect the most vulnerable of all — infants, the elderly, and people with weakened immune systems — who cannot benefit from the shot the way most of us can. To hear that fewer than 40 percent of us get an annual flu shot is maddening. Who wants to be blamed for fueling an epidemic and killing young children? I rest my case.

15
GET NAKED

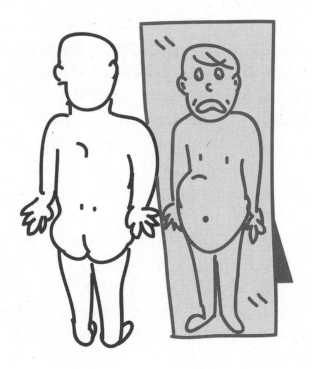

We throw our clothes on and off daily, during which time we're partially or wholly naked for a few seconds or minutes, and we spend quality time in the shower in our birthday suit. But when was the last time you took a good look at yourself butt naked in front of a mirror — front and back? You'd be surprised by how illuminating this exercise can be. You can spot trouble on the horizon in the form of body oddities that you didn't have before and signs of skin cancer. The skin acts as an indicator of the state of the entire body, and external skin discolorations, blemishes, lesions, rashes, blotches, or other unsightly marks can be signs of underlying internal disease. Once in a while, take a visual inventory of every square inch of yourself, including your hair, nails, and the inside of your mouth.

You can also get an honest sense of how well you are aging based on your physical appearance alone. Is your overall skin tone and set of wrinkles reflective of someone your age? Do you look older than your chronological age? And you can use this moment to gather measurements that can help you track the progress you're making by changing your habits. Measure your waist and see it get smaller. Start a skincare routine that nourishes the health of your skin (and keeps you examining your skin regularly). Or maybe just tell yourself that you're beautiful and doing okay. Say an affirmation as you stand there naked and accept who you are. We all know that having a strong sense of self and being comfortable in our own skin will go a long way to keeping us healthy and psychologically strong.

16
GET OFF YOUR BUTT MORE

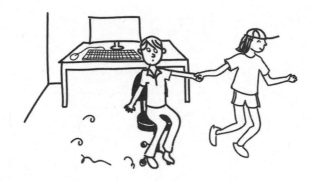

If you're a construction worker, farmer, baggage handler at the airport, or someone whose job is physically intense (in other words, you spend much of the day upright exerting yourself physically), you get a free pass on this rule and can move on to the next. But if you're like most people, you spend a great deal of time sitting as a result of your desk job, long commute, penchant for the couch, or the mere fact that you're getting older and sitting more seems inevitable. There's no end to the number of studies that prove the power of exercise in maintaining health, including a profound link between more time spent sitting and greater incidence of obesity, diabetes, cardiovascular disease, and even greater total mortality. One of the first studies ever done that pointed to the value of regular physical activity — "regular" meaning throughout the day — came out of a comparison of London's double-decker bus drivers and ticket takers in the 1950s. The ticket takers, who climbed up and down stairs all day as part of their job, had a much lower incidence of heart attacks than the bus drivers, who sat most of the day. Provocative recent studies show that physical activity even has antiaging effects on our DNA. It's true that you can change the expression of your genes — tipping the scales in favor of a long, robust life — just by getting off your bottom more. Is it any wonder that in the last century, as desk jobs became more prevalent, we witnessed a concomitant rise in illnesses related to being sedentary?

By the way, sitting itself is not the culprit here; it's the biological effects that sitting triggers in the body. Just as exercise spurs positive metabolic changes to our body, being inactive causes metabolic changes in the opposite, negative direction. And prolonged time spent sitting, *independent of how much other physical activity is done during the day,* has been shown to have significant metabolic consequences, negatively influencing such things as blood fats, cholesterol, blood sugar, resting blood pressure, and the appetite hormone leptin, all of which are risk factors for obesity, cardiovascular illness, and other chronic diseases.

Something else to keep in mind: if you think that you're doing your body good when you fit in an hour-long workout before or after a long day at your desk, think again. Even two hours of exercise a day will not compensate for spending twenty-two hours sitting on your derriere or lying in bed. No matter how much you sweat it out during a daily hardcore workout (or, God forbid, save it all for the weekend), if you're routinely sitting for hours at a time, you may as well be smoking. That's more or less the impact that prolonged sitting will have on your health risks. So get up and get moving — more! It's the only proven fountain of youth.

17
JACK YOUR HEART RATE UP 50 PERCENT ABOVE YOUR RESTING BASELINE FOR AT LEAST FIFTEEN MINUTES EVERY DAY

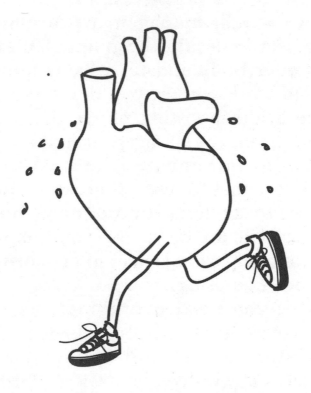

To reap the benefits of exercise, including all those biochemical reactions that take place to lower your risk of illness and keep your body humming, aim for breaking a sweat and getting your heart pumping fast for a minimum of fifteen minutes a day. We know now that the old guidelines recommending about a half hour of exercise five days a week are just that — old. If you stick with that minimum, you won't stop weight gain as you get older unless you really scale back the caloric intake. And even if you do achieve weight management through diet alone, that's beside the point. Unless you move your body and force your lungs and heart to work harder, you don't experience all the health-boosting pluses that exercise offers, from reducing your risk of heart disease to minimizing the chances that you'll become obese, diabetic, and depressed. In the long run, routinely breaking a sweat will do more for your happiness than routinely eating slices of chocolate cake (and not exercising).

And if you needed one more reason to push yourself physically, consider this: a high-intensity workout could make you smarter. On average, there are 100 billion neurons in each of our brains, and they love a good physical workout. Studies now show that older people who still do vigorous exercise, play competitive sports, or just walk several times a week protect their brains' white matter from shrinking. So if you plan to have a superbly functioning brain in your golden years, and dodge the evils of senility and Alzheimer's disease, then commit to an exercise routine. It can be as simple as leisurely walking.

18
START A SENSIBLE CAFFEINE HABIT

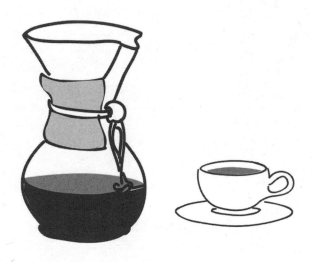

As with moderate drinking, consuming caffeine in moderation from natural sources like the coffee bean and tea leaf has long been shown to confer positive benefits on our health. Anecdotal evidence alone tells us that caffeine helps us feel energetic, alert, and upbeat. It can even help us to run faster or cycle quicker, which is why coffee is often the beverage of choice for runners and cyclists before races. This is due to caffeine's stimulating effects on the cardiovascular and central nervous systems. It prepares the brain and body for action by triggering an increase in heart rate, dilating your body's 60,000 miles of blood vessels to ease blood flow, and boosting sensitivity to stimulation. Although researchers have tried to link caffeine consumption with illnesses such as heart disease, hypertension, osteoporosis, and cancer, study after study has proven otherwise. Caffeine, especially from traditional sources and not modern, factory-made concoctions that sell as energy drinks, may actually have protective anticancer properties. But, again, moderation is key.

Too much of a good thing will turn ugly, as overconsuming caffeine can make you prone to anxiety, headaches, migraines, feeling jittery, and more. And while rare, caffeine overdosing can happen if you imbibe some of today's concentrated energy drinks. Slowly sipping a hot coffee is not the same as quickly downing a shot that's loaded with caffeine and probably sugar, too. So enjoy your coffee or tea and avoid the more processed jolts. Cut back on caffeine in the afternoon, especially after 2:00 p.m. Your body needs time to process all the caffeine so it won't infringe upon restful sleep. If you need a pick-me-up late in the day, then at least opt for tea since it has less caffeine. Or go for a walk.

19
ASK MOM OR DAD
WHAT KILLED GRANDPA
AND AUNT MARGE

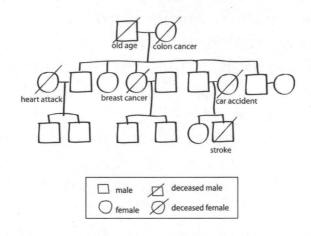

FAMILY HISTORY

□ male	◻	deceased male
○ female	⊘	deceased female

Did your grandparents die of "old age"? The last time you had to fill out a health history questionnaire in the doctor's office and you encountered questions about relatives and whether or not *anyone* in your family suffered from heart disease, dementia, or cancer, did you find yourself scratching your head? Asking our parents and other family members about the diseases in our bloodline is not an easy thing to do. But it can be more effective at helping us prevent illness than any technical test performed by a lab. In fact, family history is one of the most underused but powerful tools for understanding your health. And it's the surest way to escape more invasive tests. So buck up and ask the tough questions. All it costs is a little time questioning your relatives. Fewer than a third of families maintain a good, updated health tree, yet the Cleveland Clinic has proven that learning about your family tree is one of the best genetic tools to predict cancer risks.

If querying mom or dad and your favorite uncle over the phone sounds daunting, then make it a goal to initiate the conversation at your next family gathering. Reunions, holidays, and even funerals can make for ideal times to talk. The U.S. surgeon general operates a free website — https://family history.hhs.gov — that will help you to create a family health history and share it electronically with relatives and your doctor. One word of caution: be sure to obtain information from both sides of the family, especially if you're a woman who knows less about your paternal relatives than those from your mother's side. A higher risk for breast or ovarian cancer can originate from either side of the family.

20
CONSIDER DNA TESTING

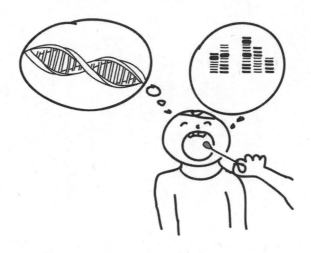

So your grandfather died of a heart attack in his fifties and your mom was diagnosed with colon cancer in her forties. What should you take from that bit of information? You might want to have your heart and colon checked out using the latest technology when you celebrate your fortieth birthday, if not sooner. The government maintains recommendations of when we all should get screened for this and that, but a much better way to know when and if you should ask for certain tests is to have an idea of your individual risks from family history. And if you wish for as much accuracy as possible, you can further add to that library of knowledge by spitting into a tube and getting your DNA screened.

Currently, we can look at genetic risk profiles for about forty conditions, from aneurysms to multiple sclerosis to stomach cancer. A small handful of companies have emerged that conduct genetic testing. I'm a firm believer in the power of this technology, which will continue to have more utility as we add more medical conditions to the existing list and learn about new associations between DNA variants and certain illnesses. The test won't only tell you what your DNA says about your risks; it can also clue you in to how your body metabolizes drugs and substances like caffeine and alcohol.

These tests do cost several hundred dollars, but once you pay for them, you'll gain access through the Internet to ongoing information relevant to you and based on new research. (Many of the companies that conduct the testing allow you to have an online account where you can keep track of new science that pertains to your unique DNA.) You'll also learn how you can modify your current behavior to reduce your risk of conditions you may be susceptible to and identify what's important to tell your doctor. In some cases, your genetic code can indicate whether you are likely to experience severe side effects from a particular drug, or whether the drug is likely to be effective, or how to dose the drug perfectly for you. By knowing how you are likely to respond to certain medications, you and your doctor can work together to make the right choices.

One of the more powerful tools that DNA screening provides is sheer motivation. I can tell you that you have a 30 percent chance of becoming obese based on the rate of obesity in the general population, which is probably white noise to you. But if your DNA could inform you that your risk of becoming obese in your lifetime is 60 to 80 percent, based on your genetics, this would likely mean something, wouldn't it? That might be enough to inspire you to pay more attention to the habits that affect your weight. Another way to look at it: if you knew that your personal risk for having a fatal heart attack in your life was 90 percent, you'd probably do everything you could to treat your heart well.

The combination of your DNA profile and the history you glean from family members can ultimately answer a lot of questions for you: Should you have a glass of wine with dinner? Should you get a mammogram before you turn forty? Can you wait until you're fifty to undergo your first colonoscopy? Is a stress test on your heart a good idea now? When should you consider taking a statin and baby aspirin? Should you be on the lookout for diabetes? Is a switch from participating in multiple marathons a year to a few half marathons a good idea given your age and risk for joint problems?

Because there is no one size fits all in medicine, it pays to be able to answer questions like these.

21
INQUIRE ABOUT STATINS IF YOU'RE OVER THE HILL

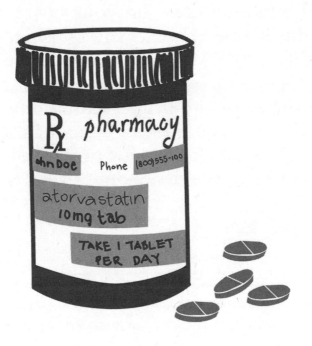

Heart disease still remains the number one killer of Americans, trailed closely by cancer and then stroke. Age-adjusted death rates from cardiovascular disease have declined 60 to 70 percent since 1950 thanks to advances in technology (including the use of statins) and better education about diet, exercise, and the risks of smoking. But the vast majority of us are still going to die of heart disease, stroke, or cancer either at a ripe old age or sooner if we don't take preventive measures. For a long time we thought statins were targeting only cholesterol, and that by reducing the body's production of cholesterol they were responsible for lowering one's risk for heart disease. But it turns out that they have a profound effect on the entire body. Statins have the power to change the whole environment by lowering inflammation — a biological process that can run amok and trigger all kinds of dysfunctions and illnesses.

To be clear, statins are compounds that inhibit a liver enzyme that plays a central role in the production of cholesterol. They are among the most commonly prescribed drugs in medicine to improve blood cholesterol levels in people who cannot control their cholesterol through diet alone, and they include such brands as Lipitor and Crestor. Statin compounds can be derived synthetically or isolated from naturally occurring foods such as red yeast rice and oyster mushrooms. But as I've already mentioned, statins don't just affect cholesterol.

When a body has high levels of inflammation markers, it means that it's encountering harmful stimuli, which can be any
number of things from germs to damaged
cells to irritants. To protect itself, the body
triggers inflammation, an elaborate response
involving the vascular system, the immune
system, and various cells within the injured
tissue. Researchers are now discovering
bridges between certain kinds of inflammation and our most pernicious degenerative
diseases, including Alzheimer's disease,
cancer, autoimmune diseases, diabetes, and
an accelerated aging process in general.
Virtually all chronic conditions have been
linked to chronic inflammation.

The first study to point out the value of
statins in reducing inflammation came out
of Harvard in 2008. It showed that taking
these drugs could dramatically lower the
risk of first-time heart attacks, strokes, and
other artery problems in healthy men over
fifty and women over sixty years of age who
do not have high cholesterol but have high
levels of inflammation markers — a sign
that something isn't right and that the body
is experiencing lots of widespread inflammation.

We know now that the real underlying
reason for cardiovascular events may not be

all about cholesterol, and that chronic inflammation is likely the cause. We also know that statins may not be all about preventing heart trouble. Since 2008, numerous other studies from impressively large controlled populations have demonstrated that statins can significantly lower our risk from dying of *anything* — cancer included. (Case in point: the *New England Journal of Medicine* published a study in 2012 involving 300,000 people that chronicled a dramatically lowered risk of death from cancer among those who took statins.)

Is a statin for everyone? Probably not. But it's worth a discussion with your doctor if you're over forty years old. In fact, pose the question as follows: "Doc, why *shouldn't* I be on a statin?"

22
TAKE A BABY ASPIRIN

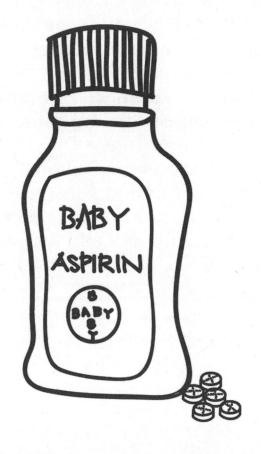

It's one of the oldest remedies known to mankind. Hippocrates, the father of modern medicine, used aspirin's active ingredient, salicylic acid, which he extracted from the bark and leaves of the willow tree, to help alleviate pain and fevers. In 1897, the German chemist Felix Hoffmann developed the first commercially available aspirin for Bayer, and since then, this wonder drug has proved its value as an effective, trusty analgesic.

Today we know that aspirin has far-reaching effects on the body as a whole that go beyond easing our headaches and sore backs. Many high-quality research studies have confirmed that the use of aspirin not only substantially reduces the risk of cardiovascular disease, but it can even ward off a medley of ailments through its anti-inflammatory powers. A daily low-dose aspirin (75 milligrams; similar to the more commonly available dose in the United States of 81 milligrams) has even been shown to reduce the risk of developing common malignant cancers in the lungs, colon, and prostate by a staggering 46 percent. So if you're basking in the glory of middle age, this might be something you'll want to discuss with your doctor (as there are side effects to aspirin such as bleeding that are real). It's the cheapest fountain of youth around and requires no prescription.

23

ABIDE BY SCREENING AND BOOSTER VACCINATION RECOMMENDATIONS

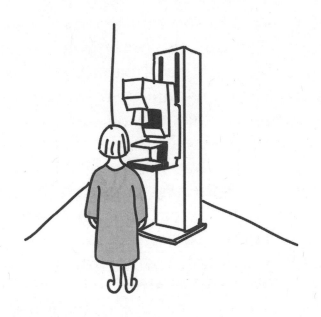

When our children are born, we take them to the pediatrician like clockwork for their regular checkups, and we (and the government) insist on vaccinating them for the measles, mumps, rubella, and polio. Why? Because we know these preventive strategies save lives. But as adults, we tend to get lazy and cavalier about keeping up with our own screenings and receiving booster shots. But this allows you to take advantage of the power of preventive medicine.

If you consider the major cancer killers in men, the top three are prostate, lung, and colon cancer. Together they represent almost 60 percent of deaths from cancer. If you're a man, prostate specific antigen (PSA) tests can identify prostate cancer early through a simple blood sample. If the subsequent prostate biopsy reveals that you have a form of high-risk prostate cancer, then you may benefit from treatment, whether that means surgery or radiation therapy. In the case of lung cancer, giving up cigarettes and minimizing your exposure to secondhand smoke can certainly decrease your risk for this type of cancer, and chest CT screenings can further decrease your chance of death from this disease. Colon cancer can similarly be avoided through colonoscopies that identify and remove polyps prior to their becoming cancerous. If you're a woman, the top cancer killers are those of the breast, lung, and colon. Again, you can help prevent and treat all of these with current screening tools, which have a profound impact on your chances of ever dying from these diseases.

Whether you're a man or a woman, preventing or delaying heart disease and stroke is also relatively straightforward and doable. We now know how certain dietary rules and the use of statins and baby aspirin, where appropriate, can come into play. You can also undergo a stress test for your heart, among other readily available tests, if you're at high risk for heart disease.

And don't forget about your booster shots and adult vaccines. Science has developed a panoply of new vaccines that weren't available to our parents, and they can help us to avoid things like whooping cough, shingles, certain kinds of pneumonia, and hepatitis B. Of course, your age and risk factors will determine when and if you need them. But ask! And if you're a parent of a teenager, inquire about the vaccine against the human papillomavirus (HPV). Immunizing your adolescent against this ubiquitous virus will help dramatically reduce his or her lifetime risk of various cancers.

24
PLAN A ONE-, FIVE-, TEN-, AND TWENTY-YEAR HEALTH STRATEGY

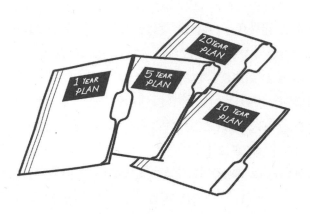

We all need goals. They help us to stay focused and give us something to look forward to. It's common to create goals for our professional pursuits and personal dreams such as buying a home and starting a family. But what about those other goals that have everything to do with our longevity and, let's face it, our ability to achieve *any* goal. Granted, lots of people resolve to lose weight every year, but that goal eludes most people. It's hard to lose weight when the weight goal is specific but the plan is not. Better to design a one-, five-, ten-, and twenty-year health strategy. Where do you see yourself in twenty years from a health perspective? What will you look like if you keep on the same path you're on now? What do you *want* to look like? It's hard to picture ourselves that far in the future, but it can help inform the choices we make today. So devise a plan and then work backward. Come up with little milestones you can achieve on that path. Instead of saying, "I will lose weight," reframe that goal to include the measures you'll take to get there. For example, "I will work out at least five days a week for thirty minutes at a time"; "I will remove 80 percent of processed foods from my diet"; "I will see my doctor once a year for a routine checkup."

As you think about where you want to be in a year, and then in five, ten, and twenty years, consider more than just your physical looks (although that's often a telltale sign of overall health and wellness). Reflect on your entire family while you're at it. Will you be able to keep up with your kids (and possibly grandkids) two decades from now? What steps can you take to ensure that you're able to take care of your spouse, who already has a chronic condition today? In five years, which risk factors will you need to pay extra attention to, given your age then? And in ten years, if you could look back to today, what would you want to do differently?

25
DEAL WITH SICKNESS SMARTLY

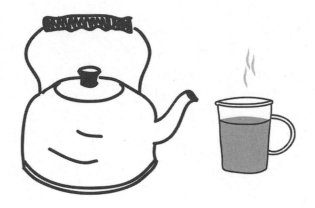

We all do it: cuddle up in bed with the shades drawn when we're nursing a bad cold or stomach virus. But part of the art of dealing with sickness means sticking to our routines as much as possible. Lying in bed all day in the dark might not be what's best for us if we want a quick recovery. Our lymph system, after all, plays a big part in fighting infections, but it won't send out its germ-fighting troops unless the body is mobile. So walk around when you're under

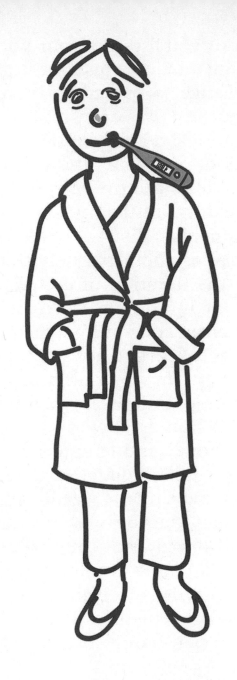

the weather. Keep your body's internal
clock on time by exposing it to the daylight;
avoid creating a nighttime setting when the

sun is out or you'll throw your body's circadian rhythm out of whack and give it another challenge to overcome in addition to illness.

When you feel a cold coming on (say, the beginnings of a scratchy throat), start sucking on zinc lozenges (more specifically, zinc acetate, the form of the metal most effective at fighting colds). Zinc — not echinacea or vitamin C — is about the only thing proven to reduce the duration of a cold. Let them melt in your mouth; they won't be of any use if you chew and swallow them. The zinc needs to be absorbed by your oral blood vessels. Shoot for 75 milligrams a day — roughly one lozenge every few hours. And drink warm liquids such as herbal teas or water with honey and lemon. The sweetness and acidity can stimulate salivation to clear your throat and sinuses. Warm drinks soothe the mucous membranes in your nose, mouth, and throat, reducing irritation.

If you think you're coming down with the flu, call your doctor right away and ask about antiviral remedies that can help you gain the upper hand sooner rather than later.

26
MANAGE CHRONIC CONDITIONS

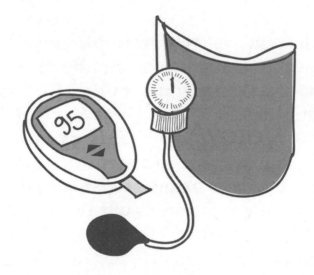

This is big. You don't want to wait until things get bad. It's so much easier to head off chronic conditions at the pass, because many are not reversible. But you can't proactively care for your body unless you undergo the blood tests and screenings appropriate for your age and history. We also have vaccines to help prevent a variety of illnesses, including ones common in later years such as shingles.

If, God forbid, you do end up having to manage something — whether temporarily or for the rest of your life — then don't slack off. Stay on top of it. This is when the severity of your condition probably dictates how well you respect its demands. For example, if you're a type-1 diabetic who relies on daily insulin just to survive, then you know you have to control your condition to a T. If you're someone with borderline type-2 diabetes whose symptoms are relatively silent, you might not be as careful, since you're not in the red zone yet. But the consequences of being so cavalier about any developing condition could be devastating, and costly.

I should add that just because we have a ton of drugs and therapies now to treat many conditions, that doesn't mean you'll want to end up having to rely on them just to live. Being drug dependent is often the result of negligence. Learn to master the management of your conditions so you help prevent or slow down their progression. In some cases, you may even be able to reverse or eliminate them entirely. Take heart from the fact that the presence of a particular condition alone can be a wonderful reminder to engage in healthy living in every area of your life, including those that have nothing to do with your illness.

27
PARTNER WITH YOUR DOC

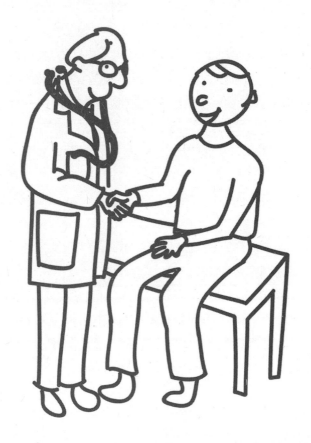

Prevention — not treatment once illness has begun — is key to optimal health and longevity. So if you haven't seen your doctor for a checkup (a quick office visit to deal with a passing cold or stomach bug doesn't count), then schedule an appointment and plan to have a comprehensive examination including any testing, vaccinations, and screenings that are relevant given your age and history.

The knowledge you bring to your doctor is more essential than your doctor's knowledge. Unfortunately, the economics of twenty-first-century medicine means that more and more physicians spend less and less time with patients. It's up to you to maximize that time. Don't assume your doctor is going to ask you every possible question to arrive at every potential solution to your concerns now and in the future. Many signs and symptoms you experience can be noted by you before you reach the doctor's office. Some people pay attention to every detail of their stock portfolio on a daily basis but not to themselves. Why not? We want quick fixes, I know. We are overloaded with information. We can feel so overwhelmed by our obligations and commitments that we end up wanting to trust someone else to make our health decisions, such as our doctor. But I'm here to tell you, this won't keep you on the best path to health.

I also recommend that you bring a friend or family member with you when you visit the doctor. It creates more accountability; you also have another set of ears. Many of us aren't in an ideal frame of mind when we're in the doctor's office, especially when something is wrong, so having someone else there can make the whole visit more bearable — and you'll remember details that you might otherwise forget. Alternatively, bring a device that can record what you hear. Many smart phones today come with a recording feature, or you can download an app to turn your phone into a voice recorder.

Modern medicine is finally moving away from the traditional "doctor knows best" paternalistic mode of decision making, in which health-care providers make key decisions for their patients. This type of decision making is slowly giving way to what we call "informed choice" or "shared decision making," in which the patient makes the final decision based on his or her goals, value system, and tolerance for risk.

A lot of decisions made in medicine today are based on someone's value system, so be sure that your opinions and convictions are respected. There's rarely a single "right" decision for treating a particular stage in a disease. The right decision for you will be the one you and your doctor arrive at together, whether it entails observation, drugs, surgery, or a combination thereof. So if you cannot speak candidly and comfortably with your doctor, find another doctor.

28
STRENGTHEN YOUR CORE AND MAINTAIN GOOD POSTURE

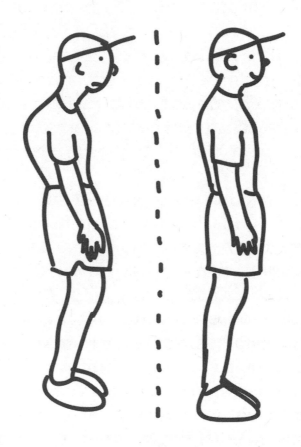

You can tell a lot about someone just by looking at the way he carries himself. Is he hunched over like an old person? Does he slouch with his head down as if he is depressed? Or is he walking fully erect, chest up, as if he is ready to take on the world with a smile on his face? With the right posture, anyone can appear younger, thinner, and more confident. But these effects aren't just for vanity's sake. Maintaining correct posture may be one of the best-kept secrets for achieving a longer, healthier, and more enjoyable life. We know that poor posture can lead to a wide assortment of neck and back problems. It is often caused by a weak core, which is one of the primary risk factors for back problems — at every age. Poor posture can also cause headaches, TMJ, arthritis, poor circulation, muscle aches, difficulty breathing, indigestion, constipation, joint stiffness, fatigue, neurological problems, and poor physical function in general.

But the risks don't end there. It's well documented that people with what's called hyperkyphosis — a posture that's hunched over, with the head and shoulders rolled forward — are 2 times more likely to die from pulmonary problems and 2.4 times more likely to die from atherosclerosis (a disorder characterized by a narrowing and hardening of the arteries due to plaque buildup) than those with normal posture.

What's more, these individuals are 1.44 times more likely to die of any cause than those with healthy posture. Even people with a mild degree of hyperkyphosis are likely to die sooner.

Bear in mind that posture also plays into our emotional state. Because posture is often linked to our facial expressions, it can subconsciously drive our emotions: when we stand tall and erect, we exude confidence. This in turn helps us to feel good about ourselves and have an optimistic outlook. All roads to perfect posture start with a sturdy core. You don't need a chiseled six-pack, but engage in exercises that work this area.

29
SMILE

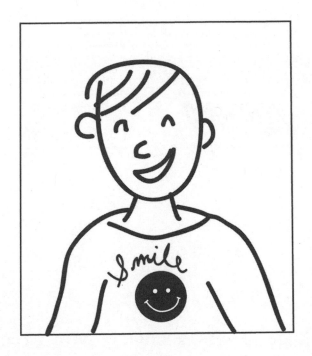

(Hint: Smiling will boost your mood no matter what. The act itself will trigger the release of pain-killing, brain-happy endorphins and serotonin. Besides, it's easier to smile; it takes seventeen muscles to smile and forty-three to frown.)

Maybe laugh a little, too.

30
Pursue Your Passions

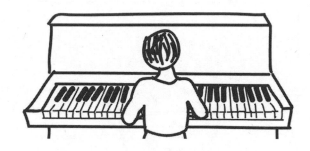

In college, I was a rower. More recently (several years beyond twenty-something), I've picked up tennis, horseback riding, and yoga. I love switching my hobbies around as I age so that I keep myself enthusiastically in the game while I also honor my body's changes through the decades. A lot of my hobbies today revolve around my kids, and my pursuits will continue to evolve as they grow older and I, of course, experience changes with the passage of time. It's important that we all develop hobbies that fulfill us in many ways — from the body's physical needs to move and play to our emotional needs to connect with other people and enjoy sports. If you were an endurance runner in your youth, you might find it hard to keep that up as you reach middle age, and you would do well to take up a new sport that's far less abusive to your knees and joints. The key is not to give up. Find a new hobby, or start learning to play an instrument, cook, garden, or pursue another passion that affords you the same rewards and will last for a while. Just be sure to choose activities that won't be abandoned quickly or that aren't highly impractical. Rather than trying to become a skydiver at seventy, for instance, check out your local Pilates studio or join a dance class at your community rec center.

31
BE POSITIVE

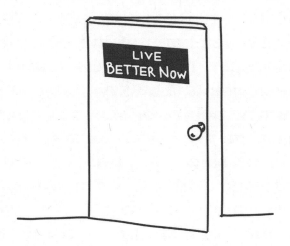

I'm a firm believer that hope and optimism are powerful forces in our lives. As with so many things, how we think determines what we experience — good or bad. And nowhere is this truer than with our health. Whether or not we have faith in our health has everything to do with whether or not we have a healthy body. If we believe we can be healthier, guess what: we will be.

Some of the most dramatic experiments putting this idea to the test are those in which people unknowingly receive fake (placebo) treatments for real health problems and come out reporting that they have improved just as much as those who got the real treatment. The placebo effect is all about a positive belief system. On the other side of the equation are stories that reveal the power of a negative belief system, one of which was famously documented in 1974 when Sam Londe was diagnosed with esophageal cancer. At the time such a diagnosis was a death sentence, so no one was surprised when he died a few weeks later, despite treatment. But what shocked the medical community was the discovery upon autopsy that Sam didn't have esophageal cancer at all. Did *thinking* that he had terminal cancer cause his premature death?

Whether or not that legendary story is in fact true down to every detail is still up for debate, but it's similar to other anecdotal evidence pointing to the power of thought. I myself notice a dramatic difference in patients' prognoses between those who believe in themselves and those who don't. In general, people who approach their life optimistically do better in clinical trials. If you believe that you are on the decline and will suffer and soon die, you may very well become a victim of such a self-fulfilling prophecy. By the same token, if you believe that you can beat the odds and enjoy a long life, you just might.

There are many ways you can boost your positive outlook. Organized, deistic religions can achieve this, but so can secular belief systems. All you need is a system that helps you to put even indescribable suffering into a wider context and tap into a higher awareness of yourself. Such a system also facilitates your sense of community and connection to other people, which is healing in itself.

32
FIND OUT WHAT EXERCISE OR ACTIVITY YOU'RE BAD AT AND FOCUS ON IT

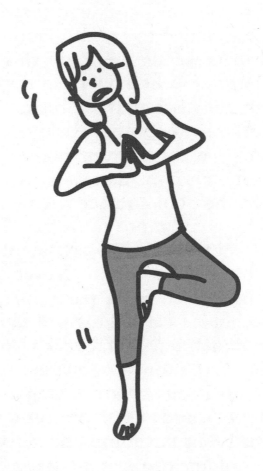

There is always room for improvement. I'm not asking you to force yourself to do anything that you truly loathe or that is completely unmotivating, but you'd be surprised by what you can discover if you try something outside your normal comfort zone. This will simultaneously challenge your body and brain in ways that can be healthful. We tend to stick with activities that we're used to doing, and that the body is well conditioned to handle. But new challenges can make us mentally sharper and physically fitter. When we push ourselves to engage in activities that we're not used to, we effectively force our brains to think harder and we compel our bodies to adapt to different circumstances. Bad at swimming? Hit the pool and see if you can swim a few laps today, more tomorrow. This will stimulate your body and work latent muscles that are hungry for action. Never cooked a meal from scratch for a party of ten? Sign up for a cooking class. This will tap creative areas of your brain that you haven't flexed in a while. Can't touch your toes or balance on one foot? Focus on stretching more (and see Rule 44) and work on your balance. You'll need that flexibility and sense of balance the older you get to keep up with normal activities. By identifying activities that you're bad at, you can improve your body's weak spots and at the same time find fun, engaging hobbies that you may grow to love.

33
PROTECT YOUR EYES AND EARS

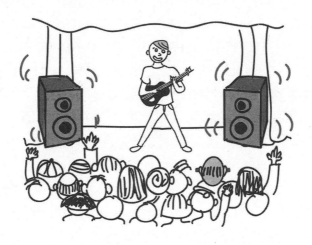

Most of us take our senses for granted if they are alive and well. But we don't realize how much our quality of life hinges on those senses — being able to hear, touch, taste, smell, and see. And many of us have at least one or two senses in particular from which we derive a lot of pleasure and/or profit. Think of the surgeon who needs his eyesight and sense of touch to execute his skill. Or the chef who relies on her sense of taste and smell to craft award-winning meals. The composer who depends on his ears to hear the notes and his hands to feel the instrument he plays. Losing your senses is not necessarily inevitable if you protect them over time and keep track of any changes so you can discuss them with your doctor. This is especially true when it comes to your eyes and ears — two senses that can be directly impacted by the way you choose live.

While we can't do anything about the loud rock concerts we attended in our youth or the days we didn't wear sunglasses while outside, we can do better going forward. Do you watch the volume on your headphones as you listen to music? Do you protect your eyes while enjoying the sun? The longer you can keep your eyes clear and your ears sensitive to sound, the longer you can enjoy seeing and hearing without medical intervention.

34
DON'T FORGET YOUR TEETH AND FEET

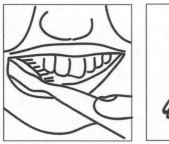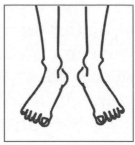

Many years ago, some researchers claimed that gum disease could lead to heart disease. While the two may not sound related, scientists believe that the heart can be weakened by agents in the blood that respond to inflammation, and chronic gum disease produces constant inflammation. So flossing at least once a day is a good idea. Not only will it go a long way toward protecting your teeth and gums (and lowering your body's overall inflammation), it's also just plain old good hygiene.

There's no serious science to prove that

one of the biggest regrets of older folks is that they failed to take care of their teeth and feet when they were young. But large surveys and personal accounts from people who spend a lot of time with the elderly tell us this is so. If allowed to deteriorate, teeth and feet will cause misery. Poor oral hygiene can produce terrible tooth decay or, worse, the total loss of teeth; not taking care of your feet can result in painful bunions, corns, warts, and other podiatric torments that make walking difficult, if not impossible. What's more, the feet contain thousands of receptors that help you to gain information about your whereabouts — literally. Many of these receptors contribute to your sense of balance and ability to walk. A whopping one-quarter of the bones in the body are located in the feet, demonstrating their complexity. And let's not forget that together, our teeth and feet are major connectors to the world around us. We use our teeth to obtain nourishment and our feet to navigate our paths through life.

So don't forget them. Visit the dentist at least once a year, twice if you've got a mouth prone to problems (your dentist can tell you that — he or she is a partner in your health care, too). Ask about proper brushing, flossing, and which toothpaste and toothbrush are best to use (and don't forget to tend to the health and hygiene of your tongue — the only muscle in the body that's attached at one end). The newer electronic toothbrushes might be worth the extra money if they prevent you from long, expensive stays in the dentist's chair getting uncomfortable dental work done. As for your feet, splurge on foot massages once in a while if that's your thing. Take note of weird-looking or painful growths or discolorations that emerge and do something about them. Buy good and comfortable shoes! Trust me, your teeth and feet will thank you later on.

35
LEARN CPR

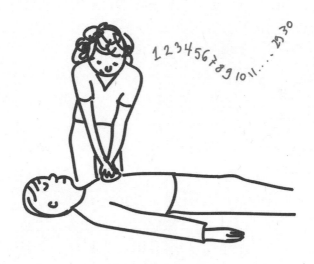

I won't teach you this lifesaving skill here, but learn it. The American Heart Association and lots of community centers conduct classes throughout the year. Sign up and get certified. You never know when you might need to use it. Best of all: most courses today (and they will take up only half a Saturday morning, if that) will teach you how to use a defibrillator, how to deal with a choking incident, and how to revive an infant who stops breathing — all excellent skills to have that don't require rigorous study, training, or even a test!

36
MAKE A MOBILE SUPPLY KIT
FOR EMERGENCIES

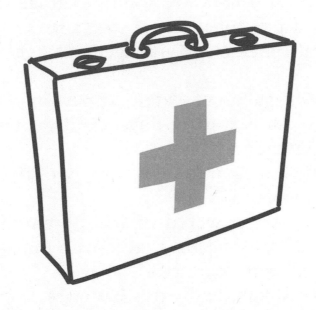

Disasters can strike at any time, anywhere. From wild weather patterns that prompt tornadoes, hurricanes, and blizzards to earthquakes, tsunamis, nuclear fallouts, and dark days like 9/11, unexpected catastrophes can be buffered by preparation. Being ready will also help you to survive a disaster and recover sooner. Have a plan with family members about where to meet if a catastrophe strikes and how to get in touch with one another (remember, your cell phone might not work, and if you don't have a way to recharge it, it may not last long).

Sites like Ready.gov can give you plenty of tips on how to prepare, including making a disaster kit. Below are some essentials you'll want to put together, as suggested by the Federal Emergency Management Agency[*]:

- One gallon of water per person per day for at least three days, for drinking and sanitation
- At least a three-day supply of nonperishable food
- Battery-powered or hand-crank radio, a NOAA weather radio with tone alert, and extra batteries
- Flashlight and extra batteries
- First aid kit
- Whistle to signal for help
- Dust mask to help filter contaminated air and plastic sheeting and duct tape to shelter in place
- Moist towelettes, garbage bags, and plastic ties for personal sanitation

[*] Adapted from the Federal Emergency Management Agency's list at www.fema.gov.

- Wrenches or pliers to turn off utilities
- Manual can opener for food
- Local maps
- Cell phone with charger, inverter, or solar charger

Additional items to consider given your circumstances:

- Prescription medications (a full week's supply) and glasses or contact lenses
- Infant formula and diapers
- Pet food and extra water for your pets
- Cash or traveler's checks and change
- Important family documents such as copies of insurance policies, identification, and bank account records in a waterproof, portable container
- Sleeping bag or warm blanket for each person. Consider additional bedding if you live in a cold climate.
- Complete change of clothing, including a long-sleeved shirt, long pants, and sturdy shoes. Consider additional clothing if you live in a cold climate.
- Household chlorine bleach and a medicine dropper. When diluted to nine parts water to one part bleach, bleach can be used as a disinfectant. Or in an emergency, you can use it to

treat drinking water by using sixteen drops of regular household liquid bleach per gallon of water. Do not use scented or color safe bleach, or bleaches with added cleaners, to treat drinking water.

- Fire extinguisher
- Matches in a waterproof container
- Feminine supplies and personal hygiene items
- Mess kits, paper cups, plates, paper towels, and plastic utensils
- Paper and pencils or pens
- Books, games, puzzles, or other activities for children

And while you're at it, throw in a copy of *The Worst-Case Scenario Survival Handbook* by Joshua Piven. That should answer any lingering questions you have when a crisis comes. Store all your emergency supplies in waterproof containers that are easy to access.

37
EAT MORE THAN
THREE SERVINGS OF
COLD-WATER FISH A WEEK

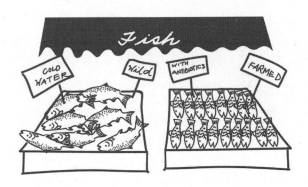

Cold-water fish, such as salmon, sardines, tuna, trout, anchovies, herring, halibut, cod, black cod, mackerel, and mahi-mahi are excellent sources of high-quality protein, healthy fats, and naturally occurring vitamins and minerals. Aim to eat cold-water fish a minimum of three times per week. The one exception: it's better to avoid fish than to consume any sea creatures that are not recommended by Seafood Watch,[*]

* For details relating to where you live, refer to

which keeps a running record of safe, ocean-friendly seafood. You'll want to skip fish high in mercury and anything from dirty waters. Wherever possible, buy wild-caught fish.

38
Eat at Least Five Servings of Fruits and Vegetables a Day

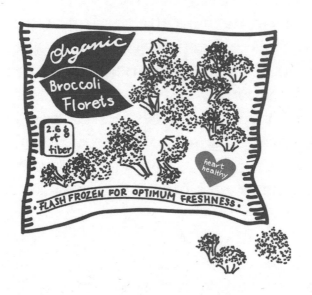

There is convincing evidence that eating at least five servings of fruits and vegetables a day can help prevent chronic diseases, not to mention decrease one's risk for obesity. But most people consume less than two cups of fruits and veggies a day, far below the four to six cups we should be getting. Think of it this way: the more fruits and veggies you consume, the less likely you'll be to replace them with nutrient-poor, health-depleting options. So eat up, and if you're going to favor one type of produce over the other, go for more leafy greens and fibrous vegetables than sugary fruit. Choose many colors, as nature segregates nutrients by color; the blend of nutrients that makes a carrot orange is different from the blend that makes broccoli green, but they both are needed to support health. To maximize the number of different nutrients you consume, you're better off eating a yellow bell pepper and a red one than eating two of a single color. Flash-frozen is fine and may actually be better than fresh (see Rule 5).

39
Speak Strongly to
the Next Generation

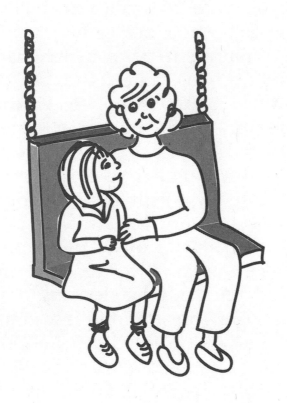

It's quite natural to feel invincible when
you're young and to shun any recommendations about how to be healthy. But when
you're young, you're setting the foundation

for your later years. So as adults, it's important that we do our best to inform and teach the next generation. The key is to find words and images that are relevant to them. Find a way to explain things to young people so that they can understand your vocabulary and jargon. While I was teaching a lesson on antioxidants to a lay audience, someone recommended that I use different colored marbles to represent types of free radicals in the body. At the time I thought it was rather goofy, but it worked. Visual imagery can be powerful and convincing, especially to younger folks.

I once had a tough time telling my kids why chocolate milk isn't the best thing for them. It wasn't until I showed them a demonstration marvelously performed by celebrity chef Jamie Oliver that they finally understood me (and heeded my advice). Jamie put sugar consumption into dramatic perspective when he filled a yellow school bus with the amount of sugar added to the Los Angeles Unified School District's flavored milk in one week. It was a visually overwhelming scene to watch as the "sugar" (in this case, white sand) rose above the windows and overtook the bus.

Some parents find it easier to talk about sex than to discuss issues with food that could touch on matters of weight or weight-related diseases like anorexia. But the sooner you establish an open communication pattern, the sooner your kids will come back to ask more questions and, believe it or not, ask for your advice. Remember, they won't accept any sage words of wisdom from an elder unless they can comprehend what's in it for them and how it will affect them. They will want to know, Why does it matter to me now? When my kids understood just how much sugar they consume thanks to Mr. Oliver's visual example, they still wanted to know why it mattered to them at that moment. That's when I had to explain that their eating habits play into how well they perform — at school and in sports. If they want to be able to think clearly, ace exams, and win important games for their team, they need to be mindful of how they are nourishing their brains and bodies. It's not always easy to make certain facts highly relevant to kids, but when you relate things to their current goals and ambitions, you have a better chance of getting them to listen.

40
EMBRACE YOUR OCD SIDE

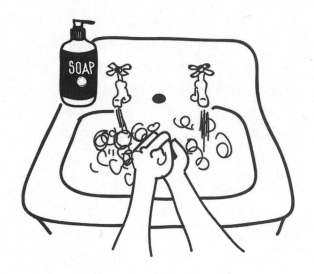

A little bit of obsessive-compulsive disorder can go a long way to keeping you healthy. You don't need to alphabetize your medicine cabinet, accumulate junk, or wear white gloves when you drive, but if you consider what OCD offers — reliable routines — you can see how it might relate to staying healthy. With a little OCD, you'll remember to wash your hands regularly, especially after exposure to germy things like bathrooms and raw chicken. You'll be strict with your daily schedule. And you'll maintain tidy living quarters that will help with your hygiene and peace of mind.

41
NEVER SKIP BREAKFAST

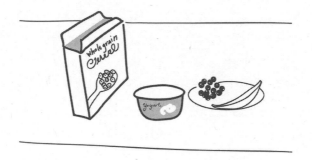

This old adage will never die. After fasting all night long, your body needs a metabolic jump-start to begin the day. We know that people who eat breakfast are just plain healthier in general and rarely have issues with weight (and if they do, the weight sloughs off once they start eating breakfast!). Skipping those morning calories to lose weight is one of the worst habits a person can develop. Front-loading your eating in the early part of the day will prevent you from overconsuming later, help you burn more calories, and allow you to get a wallop of nutrients when you need them. Moreover, eating breakfast will give your brain a much-needed boost, fueling your productivity and creativity for the entire day. If you wait too long to eat after rising, stress hormones will start pumping and sabotage your body's healthy metabolism. Too high a concentration of stress hormones like cortisol will encourage your body to retain fat, among other undesirable things.

42
SEVENTEEN MILLIGRAMS
TWICE A DAY

This rule is wholly mine. Whenever someone asks me to prescribe *something* to make
her feel better, I often joke, "Seventeen milligrams twice a day." It's my way of saying
there is no cure-all or pill that will make
you feel better. You hear about people getting vitamin B_{12} shots or vitamin infusions
and they miraculously improve. The path to
improvement is not finding the one thing
you are lacking — it's following a collection

of rules. By sticking to as many as possible, your chance of a long, fulfilling life goes up.

43
TAKE THE POSITIVE FROM GETTING A DISEASE

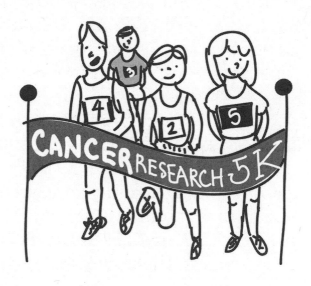

Don't throw out the rules of prevention once you've been diagnosed with an illness or medical condition. Consider such a diagnosis a wake-up call. Use the opportunity to focus on yourself and develop more long-term health strategies. Having heart disease, for instance, doesn't give you permission to eat red meat five days a week and skip exercise. Neither does it mean you earn a free pass to avoid the things you can do to prevent *other* health challenges likely brewing beneath the surface. Cancer doctors like me know that most patients who survive their cancer don't actually die of cancer in the end. They succumb to something else, usually as a result of neglecting that area of their life as they focused too much on their cancer. For example, women who survive breast cancer are more likely to die of heart disease than of cancer. So don't forget the general rules of prevention while you're managing a condition or combating a particular illness.

44
S-T-R-E-T-C-H

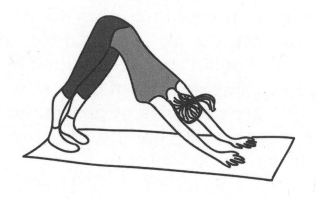

You don't have to aspire to an Olympic gymnast's flexibility, but make room for stretching exercises in your routine. This will help you to maintain the physical pliancy you need to keep up with normal day-to-day activities like getting in and out of cars, navigating your kitchen, and picking up objects. It also will help you to work on two other key skills: coordination and balance. According to the U.S. Centers for Disease Control and Prevention, one of every three Americans over the age of sixty-five falls each year, and among individuals aged sixty-five to eighty-four, falls account for 87 percent of all fractures and are the second leading cause of spinal cord and brain injury.

So in addition to your physical activities, make room for stretching. Your joints — and your inner yogi — will love it.

45
KEEP A TO-DO LIST

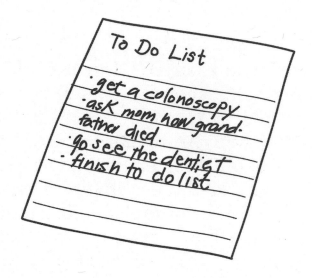

Lists are great for many things beyond shopping. They are an automatic scorecard, a way to track ourselves, and a means to hold ourselves accountable for what we want to achieve. Alongside your one-, five-, ten-, and twenty-year plans, keep a to-do list that contains those little steps and strategies that you're tackling. To-do lists can be created for all sorts of major goals, so don't limit yourself to just one long list. Maintain daily, weekly, and yearly lists. Daily to-do lists can contain your top priorities for the day, the minutes you want to spend in motion, the time you've blocked off to take a breather, and your bedtime. Weekly to-do lists might spell out the meals you want to cook, friends you want to catch up with, and the hobby you want to try or your new ideas for a workout routine. Yearly lists should include reminders for doctor visits, screening tests, and annual vaccines.

If you share your big-goal lists with family members you can count on the good ol' accountability factor to keep you motivated.

46
ASK FOR HELP

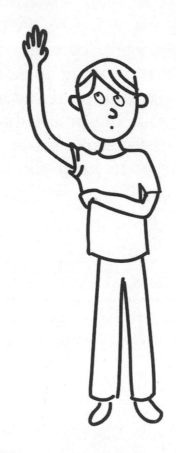

It takes a lot of courage to ask for help. We are incredibly autonomous creatures, and as Americans we especially are inclined to act independently. We prefer to solve problems on our own and value stubbornness as if it were a positive characteristic. But sometimes our challenges are just too big. Know where your limitations are, and respect them. There is nothing wrong with asking for help when the time comes, whether it's asking for support in learning how to live with diabetes, getting to the bottom of your insomnia, designing a dietary and exercise protocol that suits your needs, or finding a therapist to deal with psychological issues that are affecting your quality of life. Don't assume you can take care of everything all the time. None of us can. And none of us can be an expert in everything, even with the Internet at our fingertips. Be willing to surrender and enjoy the benefits of someone else's wisdom and experience — from professionals to friends, who can take the stress out of a concern or worry by sharing their own struggles.

47
HAVE CHILDREN

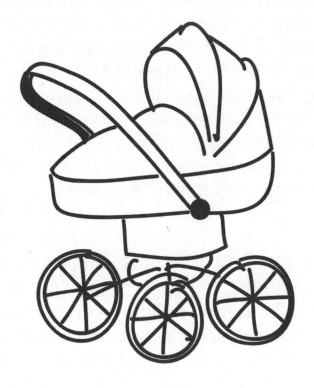

This rule won't be for everyone, but here's one reason why it's worth entertaining the idea: you'd be more likely to live longer than your childless counterparts. Seems counterintuitive because with children comes a lot of extra stress. But perhaps part of the reason people who have kids outlive those who don't is that they take better care of themselves in general and are less likely to engage in the kinds of activities that increase their risk for premature death. There's also something to be said for all that running around you do with children. The mere act of raising a child compels us to remain active and mentally challenged — both good things for health.

48
COMPLY

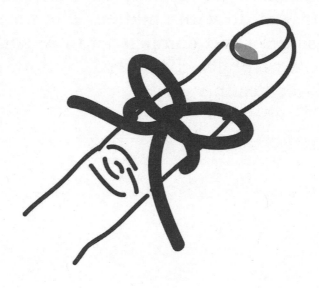

Being able to prevent, manage, and treat any condition or illness successfully hinges on being able to comply with recommended medications, including dosage (how much to take) and timing (when it's best to take it). Noncompliance is one of the biggest problems in health care today; according to a 2005 Harris Interactive report, roughly half of all prescriptions for drugs to be taken on an ongoing basis are either not completed or are never filled in the first place. Drugs that treat asymptomatic conditions, such as high blood pressure or high cholesterol, are the most likely not to be taken. Yet in the long term, the effects of not taking these medications can be devastating. The lesson: regardless of how you feel, abide by your medication's instructions as if your life depended on it, and if you don't, be honest about it with your doctor.

49
Pick Up a Pooch

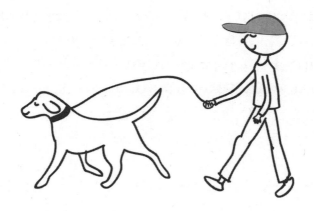

It's long been known anecdotally that dog owners are often the happiest, most upbeat people. But it's not all about the companionship of having a pooch to love and care for. Owning a dog demands that you maintain a relatively constant and reliable timetable, tending to the animal's ritualistic feedings, walks, and naps. In other words, it has the overall effect of forcing set patterns that foster health — namely sticking to a regular schedule. It also helps that walking a dog compels you to move, to engage in at least some physical exercise, even if Fido isn't a feisty greyhound looking for a run. Being outside in nature with dogs also offers the benefits of downtime, as walking dogs requires that you leave your desk and cease multitasking — other than scooping up poop and talking on your cell phone at the same time.

50
HAVE THE TOUGHEST CONVERSATION

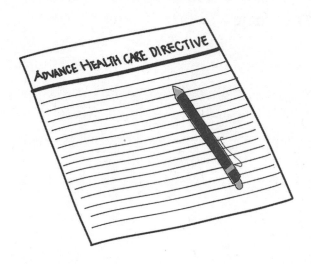

Sorry to bring you down, but this rule is typically swept under the proverbial rug until after the fact. Conversations about end-of-life decisions and life-sustaining medical treatment are not fun. But they make for far easier moments when the time comes to deal with a family crisis. There is no enjoyment in meeting doctors for the first time and coping with complex medical issues you have never encountered (or that your loved ones face when you're incapacitated). Should you become incapacitated and doctors turn to your family members for answers, they should be prepared for questions like, Do you want everything possible done to keep you alive? Nothing? If you have to go on life support, is that okay with you? Where do you want to draw the line? Who is responsible for making decisions on your behalf? Although we'd hope that our family members can agree on making decisions based on our wishes, unless things are spelled out somewhere (in a legal document such as a living will or health proxy), arguments and discord can arise quickly. So prevent that from ever happening by having a set of nonnegotiable instructions that leaves no room for doubt or disagreement.

A number of tools are available today to guide you through conveying your wishes under a worst-case scenario. A good place to start is the Prepare website (preparefor yourcare.org), designed by researchers from the San Francisco VA Medical Center and the University of California, San Francisco.

51
UNDERSTAND BASIC BIOVOCABULARY

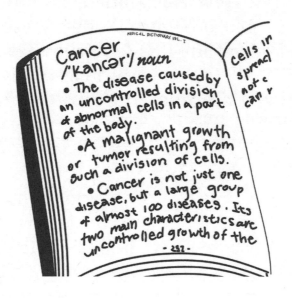

Could you define "inflammation" in a sentence or two? Do you know what "cancer" really is? How about "heart disease" and the signs of a heart attack? Do you know the difference between a "vitamin" and a "medication"? Or, for that matter, a "drug" and a "supplement"?

These are key terms everyone should understand; they crop up every day in the popular media. Read up on them so that when you come across health headlines in the news, you can understand what the article is saying and how the new research might apply to you. Think of it this way: When you shop for a car, you're knowledgeable about important lingo like what "zero to sixty" means, or how highway MPG differs from city MPG. Knowing certain definitions in the car industry allows you to make better decisions about which car to buy. The same holds true in the health industry. When you're familiar with fundamental vocabulary, you're empowered to make better decisions about your health.

52
MAKE YOUR OWN
DEFINITION OF HEALTH

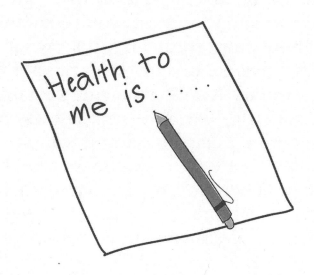

What does being healthy mean to you? Running a mile in under six minutes? Looking svelte enough to adorn the cover of a magazine? Having control of your diabetes? Avoiding the ills of your parents and living until one hundred? Everyone's definition will be different. Figure out what your personal definition of health is, and from there, develop your own code of health —

the rules you'll abide by to live up to that definition.

This entails coming up with your own set of data points, rules, or standards that say something about your health. Your weight, for instance, could be a personal metric. Your need to eat dinner by 7:00 p.m. and go to bed at exactly 9:30 p.m. to feel good the next day is also a metric. From a broader perspective, you can look at metrics as a set of habits or customs that either enhance or detract from your health.

I've given you a lot of potential metrics by which to measure your health in this part of the book. Now we'll turn to the things you would do well to avoid.

■ ■ ■ ■

PART II
WHAT TO AVOID

■ ■ ■ ■

53
BAD INGREDIENTS
AND FAD DIETS

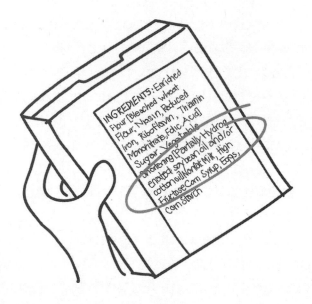

Trans fats. High-fructose corn syrup. Preservatives. Food colorings. Flavorings. Additives. MSG. Texturizers. Artificial sweeteners. Hydrolized protein. Ammonia. Fruit juice concentrate. Sodium on steroids. You know these ingredients won't win you an award for having a clean diet. Nor will foods that are known by trademarked names around the world, like Whopper, Yoplait, Cheez-It, Coke, Cinnabon, Lucky Charms, and so on. As with anything, they are fine in moderation. Remember Rule 5: Eat real food (most of the time). Real food doesn't come with a list of ingredients or claims about what it can do for you. Real food doesn't have a long shelf life and will do what living things do once they are cut from their roots or killed: it will rot.

But what about things like gluten, soy, and GMO (genetically modified organisms) that have gotten a bad rap lately? Without a doubt many people suffer from food intolerances and sensitivities and should steer clear of those ingredients that irritate their digestive systems or otherwise wreak havoc on their bodies. In large quantities, soy can disrupt the hormonal system, so moderate your consumption of it (and for the record: fermented soy that's ubiquitous in Asian cuisine is not the same as the nonfermented soy protein that is everywhere in the Western food supply). But if you eat primarily real foods, you need to worry much less about these taboo ingredients, or any others for that matter. You won't consume them in the amounts that can cause harm. Remember, too, that even products labeled "gluten free" are usually just that — products. They aren't real food.

As for GMO? Rest assured, genetically modified foods won't kill you either. GMO corn won't cause cancer, but the stress you endure while you worry about it will raise your risk. (Tidbit: We owe a lot of the hysteria around GMO to British environmentalist Mark Lynas, who was at the heart of the anti-GMO movement. In January 2013, Mr. Lynas changed his mind completely and is now a staunch GMO advocate. Why? In his words: "Well, the answer is fairly simple: I discovered science, and in the process I hope I became a better environmentalist." Amen to that.)

Speaking of science, be careful about diets that promise to cure you of everything or that have you doing weird things like taking detox supplements or undergoing liver cleanses (see the next rule). The vast majority of these diets are not backed by any scientific data and are purely profit driven. Their promoters employ lots of pseudo-science and conspiracy theories to push their agenda (and products). To some degree, diets can be helpful if they guide you to better-quality foods and teach you principles of portion control and nutrition. But there's a lot of noise out there in the diet world that tries to trump common sense and gut instinct — literally. I trust you know the difference between an apple and an apple fritter. And the great divide between a gluten-free soy burger with processed American cheese and a sirloin burger with portobello mushrooms. Which burger was made from ingredients you can actually visualize?

54
DETOXES

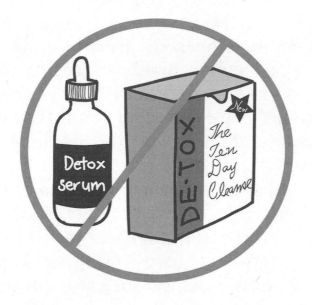

Your body is expertly designed to detox naturally thanks to your kidneys, liver, sweat glands, lungs, and digestive system. You don't need to take drastic, sometimes dangerous, measures to detoxify your body, and this includes the use of supplements and detox formulas marketed to clean you out. They are nonsense. Many of these protocols have few or no studies to back up their overpromising claims, which include reducing or removing toxins, cleansing the colon, purifying the blood, spurring weight loss, flushing fat, and treating disease. Some can be downright scary — not to mention perilous for the body. Before you even consider embarking on one of these regimes, insist on randomized studies that show these agents will produce a meaningful result. In the meantime, don't experiment on yourself before the real proof is available and widely accepted by the medical community.

We do live in a more polluted world now, but we need to be careful about accepting brash, extreme statements about the connection between toxins and possible impacts. I should point out that one of the longest-living communities on Earth — where a remarkable number of people live past one hundred — is tucked behind smoggy Los Angeles in Loma Linda. Toxins will accumulate in your body over time; it's as inevitable as the wrinkles that you'll get and the gray hair you'll grow. But there's no safe way to remove them other than relying on the body's built-in systems, which are well equipped to handle the job.

And there's no such thing as an "immune-boosting" anything. The best way to enhance your immune system is to eat well and stay active. Superfoods don't exist, either. Yes, some foods contain more nutrients than others, but it's quite hyperbolic and misleading to call any food a "superfood." Don't be fooled by anyone selling you something to "oxygenate" your body. Your lungs do that for you. Watch out for the word "cleansing," too. Your body has built-in mechanisms for that. The only things we should be cleansing are our skin, hair, teeth, and probably our garages.

55

RISKY BEHAVIORS AND DANGEROUS SPORTS

We'd like to avoid trauma as much as possible, not just for ourselves but also for our family members. Injury yields damage that tends to last a long time, if not forever. So it pays to ask yourself where and when you're willing to take risks that could have life-altering consequences.

Have you ever played or do you currently play a contact sport such as football, ice hockey, soccer, rugby, lacrosse, water polo, wrestling, boxing, or basketball? Do your kids? Contact sports don't just put you at risk for short-term injuries such as cuts, bruises, bone fractures, and pulled muscles, tendons, and ligaments. Repeated injuries, especially trauma to the head even when it doesn't cause a concussion, will have a lasting impact due to the inflammatory reactions that take place in the brain and body. This explains why so many NFL players suffer from premature heart disease and stroke while nuns win the longevity contest. It also may shed light on the shocking number of suicides among those who've suffered repeated blows to the head in contact sports, but who would not otherwise seem to be at risk of killing themselves.

Similarly, any risky behavior could shorten your life and the quality of it. These include the obvious things like smoking or drinking and driving, and they also include the not-so-obvious things like trying a triple-diamond ski run when you're a beginner or running a marathon without training. I think you know what I mean. It's one thing to challenge yourself once in a while and do something outside your normal comfort zone. But it's another thing to make a habit of thrill seeking and engaging in risky behaviors that have very obvious and known dangers. Life insurance companies don't ask you if you scuba dive or pilot a small airplane for nothing.

56
AIRPORT BACKSCATTER
X-RAY SCANNERS

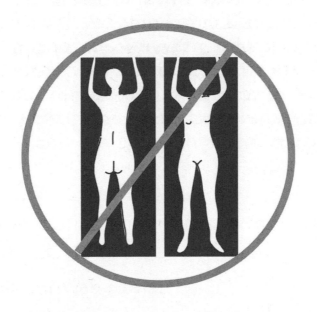

Do we really know what these machines do to us? Where's the long-term data going back decades to show they are indeed harmless? In the 1930s and '40s, shoe fitters used a type of X-ray machine called a fluoroscope to take pictures of people's feet. And guess what: those who were exposed to excessive radiation went on to develop cancers on their feet.

So until science can prove the safety of backscatter technology, I'll be requesting the manual pat-down massage when I go through the TSA's gateway at airports. You should, too. And let's campaign for better technology that doesn't entail shooting radiation through someone. (As an aside, we may be seeing these scanners gone from our airports due to all the controversy they've generated, but be aware of similar technologies that emerge without a bona fide safety history.)

57
SUNBURNS

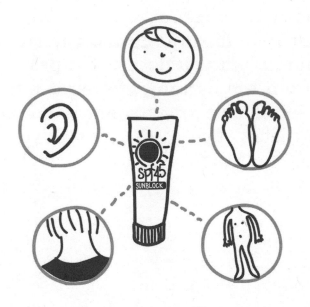

Your skin weighs approximately twice as much as your brain. It's a huge organ that acts as a barrier to protect your insides. But the fairer you are, the higher your risk for blistering sunburns. While the symptoms of sunburn are usually temporary, the skin damage is often permanent and can have serious long-term health effects, including premature aging and skin cancer. Although you shed and regrow your outer skin cells about every twenty-seven days, injury that lies hidden deep inside can manifest years later. The experience of getting a sunburn is also a lesson in inflammation, which can have a lasting impact on the body long after the burn is gone. You don't need to get a sunburn to absorb enough rays to create vitamin D, but you do need to protect your skin from the harmful effects of ultraviolet radiation. Don't forget about those hard-to-reach places such as the tops of your ears, back of your neck, and scalp (opt for a hat in that case).

58
INSOMNIA

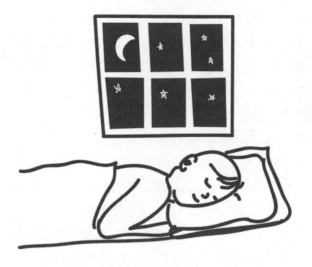

Bad nights make for bad days. We all know what lack of sleep does to us. It makes us moody, mentally foggy, unproductive, uncreative, insufferably tired, and oddly uncoordinated (some argue that serious lack of sleep is on par with drunkenness in terms of what it does to our motor skills). But those are just the obvious symptoms you probably notice. What you don't necessarily see is what's going on from a biochemical standpoint. Suffice it to say that sleep deprivation is a villain to well-being, and its antidote — restful sleep — is an unsung hero in our world. Among its proven effects, sleep can dictate how much we eat, how fat we get, whether we can fight off infections, how creative and insightful we can be, how much we can remember, how well we can learn new things, how easily we can cope with stress, and how fast we can process information. The brain is much more active at night than during the day. If you lose just one and a half hours that your body needs for one night, your daytime alertness will go down by about a third. In fact, we can make do longer without food than without sleep. The side effects of poor sleep habits are many: hypertension, confusion, memory loss, the inability to acquire new knowledge, obesity, cardiovascular disease, and depression. And when we consider the parallels between our obesity epidemic and collective sleep deprivation, we have to wonder: could sleep be the ultimate diet?

Sixty-five percent of Americans are overweight or obese, a percentage that takes on a special significance when an estimated 63 percent of American adults do not get the recommended 8 hours of sleep a night. The average adult gets 6.9 hours of sleep on weeknights and 7.5 hours on weekends, for a daily average of 7 hours. How much are you getting? Do you have fewer than 1,460 dreams a year, the average for someone who sleeps well?

For far too many people in the modern era, sleep deprivation is a badge of honor. That's why one of the first questions I ask patients who are afraid of a fatal diagnosis is simply the following: How are you sleeping?

It's no surprise that our lack of sleep has spurred an explosion in the sleep-aid industry. At least 20 percent of older American adults use some form of sleep aid, including prescription or over-the-counter drugs or even alcohol. Many use such aids every night to make them drowsy. Is taking something for sleep okay? A better question: Is this what we've come to need in contemporary society because we can't rely on our innate sleep mechanism? (And sleep is, by the way, a very natural process, like anything else our bodies do automatically for survival.)

The vast majority of people who suffer from insomnia or wakefulness during the night could find automatic, dreamy sleep again — without aids — if they identified the culprit and established a few habits to encourage 100 percent natural sleep. This means being mindful of ingredients such as caffeine that antagonize sleep if consumed too late in the day, being able to manage chronic worrisome thoughts, and being religious about going to bed at the same time every night and getting up at the same time every morning. An ideal environment for sleep is also important (for instance, no stimulating electronics in the bedroom; many of these devices emit what's called a blue light wave that will trigger wakefulness in your brain). Find a way to use sleep aids sparingly and save them for extreme circumstances such as when traveling across time zones. You may even want to take a look at which type of sleep setting is ideal for you. Are you better off in a separate bed from your spouse? Are you still trying to share a queen bed with your restless partner (who also snores)? By the age of sixty, 60 percent of men and 40 percent of women will snore during sleep. What disrupts your sleep? The number of couples choosing to sleep in separate beds or even separate rooms (upwards of 30 percent of us) isn't all that unbelievable. If you get a great night's sleep regularly, everything in life seems better, including your relationships. If you're not sleeping, there's probably a reason. Get to the bottom of it and get back those Z's. You need them.

59
STILETTOS AND OTHER SNEAKY SOURCES OF INFLAMMATION

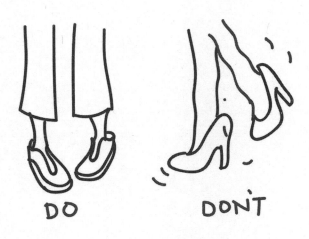

Inflammation is a normal but sometimes overactive biological response to harmful stimuli. Its ultimate goal is to initiate healing, but when inflammation becomes chronic due to disease or prolonged stress, it can become destructive. For this reason, inflammation has been linked to some of our most troubling degenerative diseases today, including heart disease, Alzheimer's disease, cancer, autoimmune diseases, diabetes, and accelerated aging.

When you're walking around barefoot or wearing uncomfortable shoes, you're causing some unnecessary inflammation in your feet that can have an impact on your entire system. If the goal is to reduce your overall inflammation and take the load off your joints and lower back to further reduce inflammation, then I know of no better, easier way to do this than to simply wear a pair of supportive and comfortable shoes daily.

Other ways to reduce sneaky sources of inflammation include maintaining a healthy weight (Rule 13), keeping a regular schedule (Rule 3), getting an annual flu shot (Rule 14), considering taking baby aspirin (Rule 22) and a statin (Rule 21), keeping a positive outlook (Rule 31), and managing any ongoing condition carefully and responsibly (Rule 26). If you have any obvious signs of chronic inflammation somewhere, be it acid reflux or back pain, take note of the condition and do what you can to resolve it.

60
JUICING

Don't think for a second that Jack LaLanne owed his longevity (he lived to be ninety-six years young) to his eponymous juicer. Perhaps he could have lived to one hundred if he had avoided this trend of pulverizing produce in a powerful blender and drinking up. Does the body really like consuming ten carrots all at once? Or a pound of radishes?

The more important question to answer is whether the original nutrients in the fruits and vegetables, which are now contained in a tall glass of juice, are in fact the same. I think not.

For starters, oxygen is a powerful oxidant. It changes the chemistry of molecules in an instant by stealing electrons. As soon as we expose the inner flesh of a fruit or vegetable to the oxygen-rich air, guess what? We oxidize it on the spot, in a fraction of a second — especially if we subject the fruit or vegetable to the disruptive power of a blender. We change its whole makeup and the nutrition that went with it. There's a reason why Tropicana sells most of its juices in nontransparent, refrigerated containers that light and air cannot penetrate. They've been in the business a long time. They know how to preserve the nutrients in their product as long as possible.

I've already stressed the importance of eating whole real foods. Juice from a juicer is not whole food — it's *processed,* because the fiber with its phytonutrients has been removed. When people say that juicing saved their health or somehow transformed their bodies, they are really saying it distracted them from eating junk food.

While the peddlers of juice drinks like to refer to all the studies about the benefits of consuming more fresh fruits and vegetables, they fail to mention that these studies don't have anything to do with juice products. They are taken from studies done on whole foods. That's like comparing apples to oranges (excuse the pun). Which means you know what you should be doing: junking the juicer and eating whole foods.

61
EATING MORE THAN THREE SERVINGS OF RED AND/OR PROCESSED MEATS A WEEK

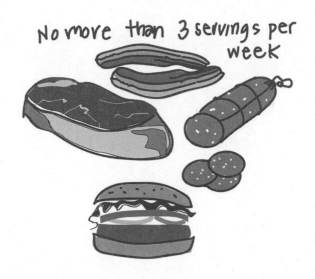

No more than 3 servings per week

As with alcohol, there are pluses and minuses to being a meat lover. The consumption of red meat in moderation isn't necessarily bad, but studies have shown that eating more than three servings a week can increase your risk for certain diseases and chronic conditions. There is also ample data that processed meats such as deli cuts, salami, ham, bacon, hot dogs, and sausages can have negative health effects. One possible explanation is that these processed meats may contain high concentrations of salt or chemicals that can be harmful. So moderate your consumption of them.

62
VITAMINS AND SUPPLEMENTS

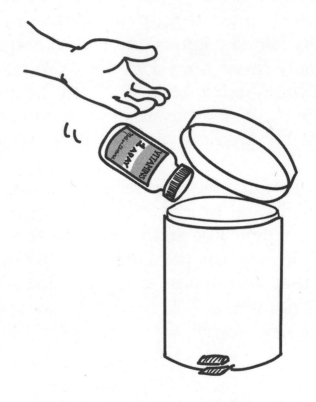

If you look at all the vitamin studies done on groups of more than a thousand people in the last few decades, many of them have shown that taking vitamin supplements is correlated with an increased risk of diseases such as cancer and produces little benefit to health. Some of these results were statistically significant, but some were not. The interactions of supplements and the body are very complex, but a simple explanation may be that the body likes to create free radicals to attack "bad" cells, including cancerous ones. If you block that mechanism by taking copious amounts of vitamins, especially those touted as antioxidants, you block your body's natural ability to control itself. You block a physiological process. You disrupt a system we don't fully understand yet.

Simply put, we cannot expect a pill or packaged food product to satisfy our nutritional needs in the same way real food can. I don't care what the label says, go for the foods that don't come with labels! And stop taking vitamins.

63 ABSENCE OF DOWNTIME

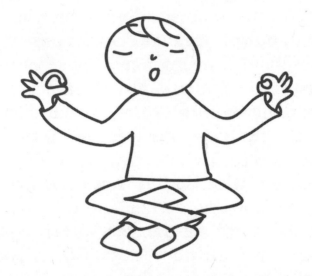

Anyone who has burned the midnight oil at work or hasn't had a restful vacation in a long time knows that a breaking point will be reached. This is when you shut down and struggle to be productive because you're just so exhausted and in need of a time-out. Too many of us try to cure our fatigue with infrequent vacations rather than scheduling downtime intermittently throughout the weeks of the year. Downtime isn't just about removing oneself from work obligations and household chores; it's also about truly relaxing in a peaceful environment in which you can let the brain take a breather and stop multitasking. This will ultimately help you to be more creative and more productive when you jump back into the game again.

Be mindful of technologies such as those found in our phones and computers, including handheld conveniences. These wondrous devices make the smallest windows of time entertaining and potentially productive. But regular use of these devices may produce an unanticipated side effect: when we keep our brains busy with digital input, we could be forfeiting downtime that could allow us to better learn and remember information, or to come up with new ideas. See if you can schedule downtime at least once or twice a week. It needn't be for long. Try a mere twenty minutes to start during which you avoid media and technology entirely and do something else pleasurable such as reading a book or going for a brisk walk (without your cell phone). Build regular downtime periods into your schedule. Your brain and body will love it.

64
SMOKING

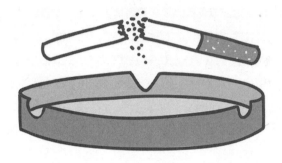

Your lungs have a lot of work to do and don't need the extra inflammation and irritation caused by tobacco. You breathe in 2,000 gallons of air a day into an organ with the surface area of a tennis court. There's enough to filter out of the air already without having to add the toxins from tobacco.

Along with being overweight, smoking is one of the most prominent risk factors in virtually all chronic illnesses. It can significantly increase your risk for all types of ailments and affect your quality of life. Anyone who quits the habit gains tremendous benefits in terms of health and longevity. While smoking can do lasting damage, the good news is that the lungs can regenerate once you stop. And it's never too late to quit smoking.

It may be legal in some places, but just because it's okay to buy and smoke marijuana doesn't make it okay for your health. We know that marijuana use can cripple the immune system and increases the risk for respiratory illnesses, cancers, and mental disorders like depression and memory defects.

65
HOARDING YOUR
MEDICAL INFORMATION

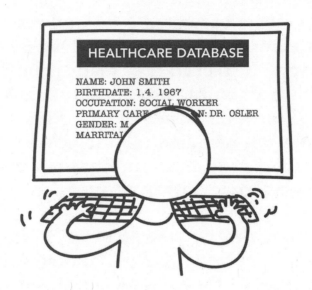

Keeping your medical information secret will do you more harm than good. You don't have to tell everyone your name, weight, cholesterol level, and what health issues you've got, but if you are given the opportunity to share your information anonymously with science (and the world at large), then do it. This will help us to build the kind of database we need to mine so we can come up with better technologies and therapies to, yes, save you and your family. This isn't about privacy. It's about giving back the raw data that we need to create new opportunities for people to live longer.

Perhaps the best way to illustrate this is to consider what happened in the fall of 2008 when Google predicted a flu outbreak three weeks before the Centers for Disease Control. How? It tracked how many people were searching for words like "fever," "chill," and "flu" and where they were. This online "sharing," in turn, led to Google's early and correct prediction as millions around the world created patterns in their online searches that could be detected and identified. Imagine the power of such an early call, which helped alert and mobilize health authorities so they could get ahead of the curve.

So share and share alike. And if your employer offers an interactive corporate wellness program, sign up!

■ ■ ■ ■

PART III
DOCTOR'S ORDERS

■ ■ ■ ■

The purpose of this section is to give you a decade-by-decade list of things to do, from the information that you should be collecting routinely about yourself to the preventive steps you can take at each age. A person in her twenties will have a slightly different to-do list than her fifty-something mother. As with all the recommendations made in this book, these are based on scientific research and follow generally accepted guidelines in the medical community.

20s

- ✔ **Blood Pressure:** Check this at least once a year or more frequently if it's previously been abnormally high or low.
- ✔ **Fasting Cholesterol:** Get your cholesterol tested after you have fasted for nine to twelve hours, which will give you a more accurate picture of your important

lipid numbers: total cholesterol, LDL and HDL cholesterol, as well as triglyceride levels. You'll want to do this test every five years or more frequently if you've had an abnormal test result.

✔ **Dental Health:** Visit a dentist annually for a checkup and professional cleaning. Go twice a year if your mouth is prone to problems like tooth decay.

✔ **Eye Health:** Visit an ophthalmologist (eye doctor) for an eye exam every two years or as your doctor recommends.

✔ **Sexual Health:** Get tested for sexually transmitted diseases; women should have an annual Pap smear and pelvic exam.

✔ **Immunizations:** Get a tetanus-diphtheria booster shot at age nineteen and the vaccine for human papillomavirus if you haven't already; get a flu vaccine every year. Individuals born in 1980 or later should receive a second varicella (chicken pox) vaccine.

✔ **Skin Exam:** Look for marks or changes on your skin monthly and have a doctor do an annual skin check.

✔ **Testicular Exam:** Perform a monthly self-exam, especially if there is a family history of testicular cancer.

✔ **Breast Exam:** Perform a monthly self-exam, especially if there is a family history of breast cancer.

✔ **Exercise:** Develop a personal exercise program and also keep track of your movement during the day with an accelerometer, and develop a daily personal activity target.

✔ **Diabetes Screening:** Have your hemoglobin A1c (also called glycosylated hemoglobin) checked if you have a family history of diabetes, a BMI greater than or equal to 25, or history of gestational diabetes. The hemoglobin A1c test will give you your average blood sugar value over the previous three months and is a better indicator of your overall number than a test that just looks at your blood-sugar value at a single moment in time.

30s

✔ **Blood Pressure:** Check this at least once a year or more frequently if it's previously been abnormally high or low.

✔ **Fasting Cholesterol:** Get your cholesterol tested every five years or more frequently if you've had an abnormal test result. A fasting cholesterol is taken after you've gone without eating for nine to twelve hours and gives a more accurate test result.

✔ **Dental Health:** Visit a dentist annually for a checkup and professional cleaning. Go twice a year if your mouth is prone to problems like tooth decay.

✔ **Eye Health:** Visit an ophthalmologist (eye doctor) for an eye exam every two years or as your doctor recommends.

✔ **Sexual Health:** Get tested for sexually transmitted diseases; women should have an annual Pap smear and pelvic exam.

✔ **Immunizations:** Maintain booster shots and get the annual flu vaccine.

✔ **Skin Exam:** Look for marks or changes on your skin monthly and have a doctor do an annual skin check.

✔ **Testicular Exam:** Perform a monthly self-exam, especially if there is a family history of testicular cancer.

✔ **Breast Exam:** Perform a monthly self-exam, especially if there is a family history of breast cancer.

✔ **Exercise:** Develop a personal exercise program and also keep track of your movement during the day with an accelerometer, and develop a daily personal activity target.

✔ **Diabetes Screening:** Have your hemoglobin A1c (also called glycosylated hemoglobin) checked if you have a family history of diabetes, a BMI greater than or equal to 25, or history of gestational diabetes. The hemoglobin A1c test will give you your average blood sugar value over the previous three months and is a better indicator of your overall number than a test that just looks at your blood-sugar value at a single moment in time.

40s

✔ **Blood Pressure:** At your doctor's office, check this at least once a year or more frequently if it's previously been abnormally high or low. At home, aim to keep tabs on your blood pressure more regularly and record your numbers. Notice any patterns that occur, such as your BP rising every afternoon or lowering after exercise.

✔ **Fasting Cholesterol and Inflammation Markers:** Get these tested every three to five years or more frequently if you've had an abnormal test result. Inflammation markers are compounds in the blood that reflect systemic inflammation going on in the body — signaling that something isn't right.

✔ **Dental Health:** Visit a dentist annually for a checkup and professional cleaning. Go twice a year if your mouth is prone to problems like tooth decay.

✔ **Eye Health:** Visit an ophthalmologist (eye doctor) for an eye exam every two years or as your doctor recommends.

✔ **Sexual Health:** Get tested for sexually transmitted diseases; women should have an annual Pap smear and pelvic exam.

✔ **Immunizations:** Maintain booster shots and get the annual flu vaccine.

✔ **Skin Exam:** Look for marks or changes on your skin monthly and have a doctor do an annual skin check.

✔ **Testicular Exam:** Perform a monthly self-exam, especially if there is a family history of testicular cancer.

✔ **Breast Exam:** Perform a monthly self-exam, especially if there is a family history of breast cancer; ask about when you should get your first mammogram. Annual mammography in this age group has been confirmed to decrease mortality but is not recommended by all professional organizations due to differing risk-benefit analyses. Options for breast cancer screening should be discussed with your provider yearly.

✔ **Exercise:** Develop a personal exercise program and also keep track of your movement during the day with an accelerometer, and develop a daily personal activity target.

✔ **Diabetes Screening:** Get your blood sugar tested at least once a year, more frequently if you've had an abnormal test result. Be sure to get your hemoglobin A1c test by age forty-five. This test will give you your average blood sugar value over the previous three months and is a better indicator of your overall number than a test that just looks at your blood-sugar value at a single moment in time.

✔ **Prostate Exam:** Get your baseline PSA test (an indicator for prostate cancer) if you're African American or there is a family history of prostate cancer; otherwise, you can wait until age fifty.

✔ **Preventive Medications:** Have the discussion with your doctor about whether a daily aspirin (75 or 81 milligrams) and statin make sense as preventive therapy based on your family history and personal risk factors.

✔ **Blood Pressure:** At your doctor's office, check this at least once a year or more frequently if it's previously been abnormally high or low. At home, aim to keep tabs on your blood pressure more regularly and record your numbers. Notice any patterns that occur, such as your BP rising every afternoon or lowering after exercise.

✔ **Fasting Cholesterol and Inflammation Markers:** Check these every three to five years or more frequently if you've had an abnormal test result.

✔ **Colorectal Exam:** Get an annual fecal occult blood testing; and consider a colonoscopy every five to ten years depending on your doctor's recommendations based on your personal risks.

✔ **Dental Health:** Visit a dentist annually for a checkup and professional cleaning. Go twice a year if your mouth is prone to problems like tooth decay.

✔ **Diabetes Screening:** Get your blood sugar tested — including the hemoglobin A1c test — at least once a year, more frequently if you've had an abnormal test result.

- **Eye Health:** Visit an ophthalmologist (eye doctor) for an eye exam every two years or as your doctor recommends.
- **Immunizations:** Maintain booster shots and get the annual flu vaccine.
- **Osteoporosis Screening:** Get a bone density test if risk factors are present. Examples of risk factors include family history of the disease, taking steroids or other certain medications, going through menopause, sedentary lifestyle, excessive alcohol consumption, tobacco use, having an eating disorder, or having had weight loss surgery.
- **Prostate Exam:** Undergo a prostate exam annually that gives you PSA values, which are indicators of prostate cancer.
- **Skin Exam:** Look for marks or changes on your skin monthly and have a doctor do an annual skin check.
- **Breast Exam:** Perform a monthly self-exam, especially if there is a family history of breast cancer; schedule routine mammography based on your risk factors.
- **Exercise:** Develop a personal exercise program and also keep track of your movement during the day with an accelerometer, and develop a daily per-

sonal activity target.

✔ **Preventive Medications:** Have the discussion with your doctor about whether a daily aspirin (75 or 81 milligrams) and statin make sense as preventive therapy based on your family history and personal risk factors.

60s

✔ **Abdominal Ultrasound:** Have this test done if you're older than age sixty-five and have smoked.

✔ **Blood Pressure:** At your doctor's office, check this at least once a year or more frequently if it's previously been abnormally high or low. At home, aim to keep tabs on your blood pressure more regularly and record your numbers. Notice any patterns that occur, such as your BP rising every afternoon or lowering after exercise.

✔ **Fasting Cholesterol and Inflammation Markers:** Check these every five years or more frequently if you've had an abnormal test result.

✔ **Colorectal Exam:** Get a colorectal exam annually. This includes, until age seventy-five: colonoscopy every ten years; fecal occult blood testing every three years with sigmoidoscopy every five years; or annual fecal occult blood testing.

✔ **Dental Health:** Visit a dentist annually for a checkup and professional cleaning. Go twice a year if your mouth is prone to problems like tooth decay.

✔ **Diabetes Screening:** Check the A1c every three years or as your doctor recommends.

✔ **Eye Health:** Visit an ophthalmologist (eye doctor) for an eye exam every two years or as your doctor recommends.

✔ **Immunizations:** Maintain booster shots and get the annual flu vaccine; get the shingles/herpes zoster vaccine once after age sixty and pneumococcal vaccine (Pneumovax) at age sixty-five.

✔ **Hearing Test:** If you are over age sixty-five, have your hearing checked.

✔ **Osteoporosis Screening:** Get a bone density test if risk factors are present and at age sixty-five for all women.

✔ **Prostate Exam:** Undergo a prostate exam annually.

✔ **Breast Exam:** Perform a monthly self-exam, especially if there is a family history of breast cancer; schedule routine mammography based on your risk factors.

- ✔ **Skin Exam:** Look for marks or changes on your skin monthly and have a doctor do an annual skin check.
- ✔ **Exercise:** Develop a personal exercise program and also keep track of your movement during the day with an accelerometer, and develop a daily personal activity target.
- ✔ **Preventive Medications:** Have the discussion with your doctor about whether a daily aspirin (75 or 81 milligrams) and statin make sense as preventive therapy based on your family history and personal risk factors.

70s and Beyond

- ✔ **Abdominal Ultrasound:** Have this test done if you've smoked.
- ✔ **Blood Pressure:** At your doctor's office, check this at least once a year or more frequently if it's previously been abnormally high or low. At home, aim to keep tabs on your blood pressure more regularly and record your numbers. Notice any patterns that occur, such as your BP rising every afternoon or lowering after exercise.
- ✔ **Fasting Cholesterol and Inflammation Markers:** Check these every year

or more frequently if you've had an abnormal test result.

✔ **Colorectal Exam:** Get an annual fecal occult blood testing; and consider a colonoscopy every five to ten years depending on your doctor's recommendations based on your personal risks.

✔ **Dental Health:** Visit a dentist annually for a checkup and professional cleaning. Go twice a year if your mouth is prone to problems like tooth decay.

✔ **Diabetes Screening:** Check the A1c every three years or as your doctor recommends.

✔ **Eye Health:** Visit an ophthalmologist (eye doctor) for an eye exam every two years or as your doctor recommends.

✔ **Immunizations:** Maintain booster shots and the annual flu vaccine; get the pneumococcal vaccine after age sixty-five if you didn't get it in your sixties.

✔ **Hearing Test:** If you are experiencing hearing loss, get your hearing checked.

✔ **Prostate Exam:** Undergo a prostate exam annually.

✔ **Breast Exam:** Perform a monthly self-exam, especially if there is a family history of breast cancer; schedule routine mammography based on your risk factors.

✔ **Skin Exam:** Look for marks or changes on your skin monthly and have a doctor do an annual skin check.

✔ **Exercise:** Develop a personal exercise program and also keep track of your movement during the day with an accelerometer, and develop a daily personal activity target.

✔ **Preventive Medications:** Have the discussion with your doctor about whether a daily aspirin (75 or 81 milligrams) and statin make sense as preventive therapy based on your family history and personal risk factors.

Health Lists

Below are some fun health lists I've put together and some that I've compiled from various readily available sources. They are the ultimate cheat sheet and will help you to remember key facts, rules, and ideas.

Regardless of age, the most important things you can do to stay healthy are:

✔ Have an annual physical exam. Find a doctor and make an appointment the same time every year for a general health check. Most people, especially if they are young and healthy, typically don't see a doctor for an annual check. Getting regular checks, preventative screening tests, and immunizations are among the most important things you can do to stay healthy. Take a personal health inventory questionnaire like the one available at my website (http://davidagus.com/hq) and bring the answers to your doctor's office.

✔ Know your family history. Family history is one of the most underused but extremely powerful tools for understanding your health. Family history affects your level of risk for cancer, diabetes, heart disease, and stroke, among other illnesses. It all starts with a conversation, so talk to your family members and keep a close eye out for any illnesses that a direct relative has experienced.

✔ Don't smoke. If you do smoke, stop! Compared to nonsmokers, men who smoke are about twenty-three times more likely to develop lung cancer. Smoking causes about 90 percent of lung cancer deaths and doubles your risk of heart disease.

✔ Be physically active. If you are not already physically active, start small and work up to a minimum of thirty minutes of moderate aerobic activity most days of the week. Also move during the day while at work and when you are engaged in other activities. Long periods of sitting raise the risk for disease. Everything counts — take the stairs instead of the elevator, go for a twenty-minute walk during your lunch break, and park on the far side of the lot at the store.

✔ Keep it regular. As best you can, you should eat, sleep, and exercise at the same time each day.

✔ Know your body. You should record every sign and symptom you experience and discuss them with your doctor.

✔ Eat a healthy diet. Fill up with fruits, vegetables, and whole grains and choose healthy proteins like lean meats, poultry, fish, beans, and nuts. Eat foods low in processed fats, salt, and added sugars. Moderation is key!

✔ Stay at a healthy weight. Balance calories from foods and beverages with calories you burn off by physical activity. Only 33 percent of adults are at a healthy weight for their height. Obesity and being overweight pose a major risk for chronic diseases, including type-2 diabetes, cardiovascular disease, hypertension, stroke, and certain cancers.

✔ Manage your stress. Stress, particularly long-term stress, can be a factor in the onset or worsening of ill health. Managing your stress is essential to your health and well-being; take a timeout each day and go for a walk or do something you find relaxing.

✔ Drink alcohol only in moderation. Alcohol can be part of a healthy, balanced diet, but only if consumed in moderation. This means no more than two drinks a day for men, and one drink a day for women (a standard drink is one 12-ounce bottle of beer or wine cooler, one 5-ounce glass of wine, or 1.5 ounces of 80-proof distilled spirits).

✔ Sleep well. The quality of your sleep can dictate how much you eat, how fast your metabolism runs, how fat or thin you are, how well you can fight off infections, and how well you can cope with stress. Keep a regular pattern of sleep; going to bed and waking up at roughly the same time is key.

✔ Avoid all vitamins and supplements. These should be avoided unless your physician tells you they are necessary.

✔ Discuss the role of aspirin and statins. Ask your doctor about using these preventive medications if you are forty or older.

Top 10 Actions to Reduce Your Risk for Illness

Taking these actions today can reduce your risk of becoming sick, especially for the two most dreaded diseases in later life: cancer and dementia.

1. Eat real food on a regular schedule.
2. Avoid vitamins and supplements.
3. Discuss aspirin and statins with your doctor when you are staring at age forty.
4. Follow the prescribed cancer screening schedules.
5. Exercise regularly and move during the day.
6. Maintain a healthy weight.
7. Avoid tobacco products.
8. Avoid direct sun exposure without sunscreen.
9. Avoid sources of inflammation.
10. Get a yearly flu shot.

Top 10 Things to Help Educate Kids About Health and Wellness

1. Explain why. All too often we just

tell our children what to do without explaining the reasons. If you don't understand why, find out.

2. Watch the Jamie Oliver videos and TED Talk about children and nutrition. You can access Jamie's videos at http://www.youtube.com/user/ JamieOliver.

3. Be a good example.

4. Encourage activity.

5. Teach them the importance of digital-free downtime.

6. Vaccines, vaccines, vaccines.

7. Take them food shopping and to the farmers market and engage them in the kitchen when you're cooking.

8. If there is an illness in the family, empower children to play a role. Put together a fund-raiser, educate others, or develop a plan for the child to help the affected person.

9. Prepare them for pediatrician visits by having them review themselves. Go head to toe and do an inventory to see if anything hurts or has changed. Encourage them to make a list of questions for their doctor.

10. Let them keep their list of medical data: weight and height over the

years, immunization records, list of hospitalizations, etc. They will soon develop the attitude that they do have a role in their health care. Allow them to have private time with their doctor.

Top 10 Causes of Death in the United States*

1. Heart disease: 597,689 deaths
2. Cancer: 574,743 deaths
3. Chronic lower respiratory diseases: 138,080 deaths
4. Stroke (cerebrovascular diseases): 129,476 deaths
5. Accidents (unintentional injuries): 120,859 deaths
6. Alzheimer's disease: 83,494 deaths
7. Diabetes: 69,071 deaths
8. Nephritis, nephrotic syndrome, and nephrosis: 50,476 deaths
9. Influenza and pneumonia: 50,097 deaths
10. Intentional self-harm (suicide): 38,364 deaths

* Data from the Centers for Disease Control and Prevention expressed as deaths in the United States for the 2010 calendar year.

Top 10 Causes of Death Worldwide[**]

1. Ischemic heart disease: 7.25 million deaths (12.8 percent of deaths)
2. Stroke and other cerebrovascular disease: 6.15 million deaths (10.8%)
3. Lower respiratory infections: 3.46 million deaths (6.1%)
4. Chronic obstructive pulmonary disease: 3.28 million deaths (5.8%)
5. Diarrheal diseases: 2.46 million deaths (4.3%)
6. HIV/AIDS: 1.78 million deaths (3.1%)
7. Trachea, bronchus, and lung cancers: 1.39 million deaths (2.4%)
8. Tuberculosis: 1.34 million deaths (2.4%)
9. Diabetes mellitus: 1.26 million deaths (2.2%)
10. Road traffic accidents: 1.21 million deaths (2.1%)

[**] Data from the World Health Organization on worldwide deaths for the 2008 calendar year.

Popular Weight Loss Myths[*]

- A little goes a long way. You can walk your way to weight loss. Truth: It takes effort to lose weight. You need more than a brisk walk a day to take — and keep — the weight off.
- Only realistic goals will help you to lose weight. Truth: You can set a preposterous goal and still make headway with weight loss.
- If you're overly ambitious with your weight loss efforts, you will fail. Truth: You can be as ambitious as you want despite the frustrations; it might keep you going.
- If you're not mentally ready to change your diet, you won't succeed. Truth: This is when just a little bit of motivation can really go a long way. If your mind is somewhat willing to make a few dietary shifts, you can succeed.
- If you lose weight fast, it won't last. Truth: Slow and steady doesn't always work. For some, fast weight loss can lead to lasting results.

[*] Source: http://www.nejm.org/doi/full/10.1056/NEJMsa1208051

Top 10 Foods High in Trans Fat[*]

1. Margarine, shortening, and other processed spreads
2. Packaged baking mixes (cake mixes, Bisquick)
3. Prepared soups (especially ramen noodles, soup cups)
4. Fast food (especially fried foods)
5. Frozen foods (products such as frozen pies, pot pies, waffles, pizzas, breaded fish sticks)
6. Baked goods (especially commercially baked products such as cakes and donuts)
7. Chips and crackers
8. Breakfast food (items like cereals and energy bars)
9. Cookies and candy (especially those that are cream filled)
10. Toppings and dips (products like nondairy creamers, flavored coffees, gravies, and salad dressings)

[*] Source: http://www.webmd.com/diet/features/top-10-foods-with-trans-fats?page=3

Top 10 Most Sugary Foods[**]

1. Granulated sugar and other sweeteners (brown sugar, honey, molasses, sorghum syrup)
2. Drink powders and soft drinks
3. Candies and nougat
4. Dried fruits
5. Cookies, cakes, and pies
6. Spreads, jams, and preserves
7. Cereals, cereal bars, and instant oatmeal packages
8. Sauces (products like ketchup, chocolate syrup, and salad dressing)
9. Ice cream, milk shakes, café drinks
10. Canned fruit packed in syrup

Top High-Glycemic-Index Foods[*]

- Soft drinks, sports drinks, and fruit juices
- White bread, pasta, rice, and noodles (don't forget bagels, baguettes, donuts,

** Source: http://www.healthaliciousness.com/articles/high-sugar-foods.php
* Source: http://www.health.harvard.edu/news week/Glycemic_index_and_glycemic_load_for_100_ foods.htm

waffles, pancakes, rice cakes, and pizza)
- Potatoes, potato chips, and parsnips
- Pretzels, commercial crackers, and cookies
- Cake and most baked goods
- Commercial cereals (refined) and instant oatmeal
- Dates, raisins, watermelon
- Most candy

Top 11 Fish with Omega-3[**]

1. Wild Alaskan Salmon
2. Arctic Char
3. Atlantic Mackerel
4. Pacific Sardines
5. Sablefish/Black Cod from Alaska or British Columbia
6. Anchovies
7. Oysters
8. Rainbow Trout
9. Albacore Tuna from the U.S. or Canada

[**] Source: US News and World Report summary from the Environmental Defense Fund's Seafood Selector and the Monterey Bay Aquarium's Seafood Watch programs (http://health.usnews.com/health-news/diet-fitness/slideshows/best-fish)

10. Mussels
11. Pacific Halibut

Top 10 Fish with Mercury Contamination*

1. Tilefish (Gulf of Mexico)
2. Swordfish
3. Shark
4. King Mackerel
5. Bigeye Tuna
6. Orange Roughy
7. Marlin
8. Spanish Mackerel (Gulf of Mexico)
9. Grouper
10. Tuna

Top 10 Most Useful Health and Medicine Websites

(Note: this doesn't mean I agree with everything on the websites, just that they are a good sources of health information.)

1. National Institutes of Health (NIH .gov)
2. Centers for Disease Control and

* Source: US FDA website data from commercial fish 1990–2010 (http://www.fda.gov/Food/FoodborneIllnessContaminants/Metals/ucm115644.htm).

Prevention (CDC.gov)
3. American Academy of Family Physicians (familydoctor.org)
4. Office of Disease Prevention and Health Promotion (healthfinder.gov)
5. Livestrong (livestrong.org)
6. American Heart Association (americanheart.org)
7. The Mayo Clinic (MayoClinic.com)
8. National Library of Medicine (MedlinePlus.gov)
9. WebMD (WebMD.com)
10. American Cancer Society (cancer.org)

Top 5 Food Poisoning Culprits*

1. Poultry contaminated with *Campylobacter* or *Salmonella*
2. Beef and pork with the *Toxoplasma* parasite
3. Listeria in deli meats and dairy products like soft cheese
4. *Salmonella* and norovirus in multi-ingredient foods such as salads that

* Source: Centers for Disease Control and Prevention

are handled by food preparers (leafy greens are a leading source of food poisoning illnesses)

5. *Salmonella* in eggs and produce

Top 10 Reasons to Go to the ER**

1. Difficulty breathing, shortness of breath
2. Chest or upper abdominal pain or pressure
3. Fainting, sudden dizziness, or weakness
4. Changes in vision
5. Confusion or changes in mental status
6. Any sudden or severe pain
7. Uncontrolled bleeding
8. Severe or persistent vomiting or diarrhea
9. Coughing or vomiting blood
10. Suicidal or homicidal feelings

Top 10 Things to Do During Cold Season

1. Get your flu shot if you haven't already.
2. Wash your hands routinely.
3. Avoid sharing food and drinks with others.

4. Stay away from sick people.
5. Don't go to work (and avoid public places) if you're feeling ill.
6. Keep zinc lozenges on hand.
7. Avoid touching your face and eating with your hands.
8. Carry hand sanitizer.
9. Avoid stuffy rooms that have poor ventilation.
10. Keep common surface areas clean.

Top 10 Reasons to Take a Walk

1. You'll prevent weight gain and perhaps walk off weight.
2. You'll reduce your risk of cancer.
3. You'll reduce your risk of heart disease and stroke.
4. You'll reduce your risk of diabetes.
5. You'll boost brain power and inspire creativity.
6. You'll improve your mood.
7. You'll relieve stress.
8. You'll stimulate a connection with nature and encourage self-reflection.
9. You'll gain an alertness on par with that you'd get from a cup of coffee.
10. You'll live longer.

ACKNOWLEDGMENTS

As I did in my first book, I have my patients to thank, for they help me hone my message daily in my interactions with them. Thank you for allowing me to be involved with your care; you teach me daily about how the body works and remind me with every visit that my work isn't nearly complete. Medicine needs to be radically improved to assist and heal each of us. I also have to thank my critics, as their words and ideas inform my thinking and have helped me to further shape and clarify my message.

It is not just a privilege, but it is also a responsibility to educate about health. I have never been on this path alone and am indebted to many dedicated individuals. This book reflects the culmination of not just my lifetime work in the health-care industry, but also my ongoing collaboration with an expansive team. First, I have to thank my collaborator Kristin Loberg. Kristin and I have been working together for close to three years now, and when I considered putting another book together, I would have done it only with Kristin's involvement. She is an amazing partner, an insightful thinker, a remarkably talented writer, and a good friend. I would like to thank her family, Lawrence and Colin (and baby number two, who is growing during the writing of this book), for allowing me to spend precious time with her over the past years. And I have to thank and applaud Chieun Ko, whose beautiful and sometimes cheeky illustrations both simplify the book's concepts and help make health fun. A big thanks to Chi's family, Brian and Luca, for sharing her with me over the past year.

Thanks to Robert Barnett, who has expertly and caringly represented, protected, and guided me through this process. David Povich, thank you for being my loving advocate and guardian. You have both been extraordinary in looking after me.

I have been with only one publishing house in my short career as an author, and I couldn't imagine a better and more supportive environment. I wish to thank my team at Simon & Schuster, led by Priscilla Painton, whose support, faith, and skill made this book possible. Her editorial insights and practical wisdom have helped me to create a much better book. Thanks also to her fantastic team, including Michael Accordino, Suzanne Donahue, Lance Fitzgerald, Larry Hughes, Nancy Inglis, Amy Ryan, Nancy Singer, Sydney Tanigawa, and the big chief, Jonathan Karp. Thank you for putting up with me and your continued support.

I am also indebted to my team at the USC Westside Cancer Center and the Center for Applied Molecular Medicine, who enables me to be both a physician and a researcher, and to find the time to write. I want to particularly thank my fantastic assistant, Autumn, and the clinic team of Adam, Angel, Claire, Julianne, Julie, Justine, Lisa, Olga, Robin, Shelly, and Mitchell. Thank you for your loyalty and friendship and the daily care you give to the patients we are honored to treat. To the research team of Jonathan, Parag, Dan, Shannon, Paul, Kian, Kristina, and Yvonne: thank you for pushing my thinking forward and dedicating yourself to figuring out better ways to treat disease.

I also have to thank those who continue to support and inspire me on a regular basis, including Jeff Fager, Sandy Gleysteen, Gayle King, Jonathan LaPook, Chris Licht,

Norah O'Donnell, Karolyn Pearson, David Rhodes, and Charlie Rose at CBS News, who empower me to be able to educate and inform. To Dominick Anfuso, Marc Benioff, Gerald Breslauer, Eli Broad, Bill Campbell, Michael Dell, Larry Ellison, Robert Evans, Murray Gell-Mann, Al Gore, Brad Grey, Davis Guggenheim, Danny Hillis, Walter Isaacson, Peter Jacobs, Clifton Leaf, Max Nikias, Fabian Oberfeld, Howard Owens, Shimon Peres, Maury Povich, Carmen Puliafito, Bruce Ramer, Sumner Redstone, Joe Schoendorf, Dov Seidman, Bonnie Solow, Steven Spielberg, Elle Stephens, Yossi Vardi, Jay Walker, David Weissman, and Neil Young: your mentorship, friendship, and advice are truly appreciated.

Thanks to Steve Bennett and his team at AuthorBytes for their creative and dynamic website management, as well as Josh Greenstein, Amy Powell, and Karen Hermelin of Paramount Pictures for their fantastic guidance in getting people to listen to the "health" message.

Last, to my family, for their unwavering support and love; thank you, Amy, Miles, Sydney, Mom, and Dad. For several generations now one of our family's best and most quoted traditions has been to always root for one another, and I couldn't have imagined a more heartfelt cheering section than the Povich and Agus extended families. Thank you all for your support, and for spreading my mission to better medicine and our health far and wide.

ABOUT THE AUTHOR

Dr. David B. Agus is a professor of medicine and engineering at the University of Southern California Keck School of Medicine and Viterbi School of Engineering and heads USC's Westside Cancer Center and the Center for Applied Molecular Medicine. He is one of the world's leading cancer doctors, and the cofounder of two pioneering personalized medicine companies, Navigenics and Applied Proteomics. Dr. Agus is an international leader in new technologies and approaches for personalized health care and a contributor to CBS News. His first book, *The End of Illness,* became a *New York Times* #1 bestseller and was also the subject of a PBS special.

The employees of Thorndike Press hope you have enjoyed this Large Print book. All our Thorndike, Wheeler, and Kennebec Large Print titles are designed for easy reading, and all our books are made to last. Other Thorndike Press Large Print books are available at your library, through selected bookstores, or directly from us.

For information about titles, please call:
  (800) 223-1244

or visit our Web site at:
  http://gale.cengage.com/thorndike

To share your comments, please write:
  Publisher
  Thorndike Press
  10 Water St., Suite 310
  Waterville, ME 04901

ETHICS FOR THE
NEW MILLENNIUM

ETHICS FOR THE
NEW MILLENNIUM

HIS HOLINESS
THE DALAI LAMA

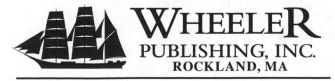

WHEELER
PUBLISHING, INC.
ROCKLAND, MA

★ AN AMERICAN COMPANY ★

Published in Large Print by arrangement with Riverhead Books, a member of Penguin Putnam Inc., in the United States and Canada.

Wheeler Large Print Book Series.

Set in 16 pt Plantin.

Library of Congress Cataloging-in-Publication Data

Bstan-'dzin-rgya-mtsho, Dalai Lama XIV, 1935-
   Ethics for the new millennium / His Holiness The Dalai Lama.
      p. (large print) cm.(Wheeler large print book series)
   ISBN 1-58724-003-3 (hardcover)
   1. Large type books. I. Title. II. Series

[BJ1012.B742 2001]   MAR 1 5 2001
294.3'.5—dc21   *CenT*

                                                        2001017517
                                                        CIP

Contents

Ethics for the New Millennium

PREFACE

Having lost my country at the age of sixteen and become a refugee at twenty-four, I have faced a great many difficulties during the course of my life. When I consider these, I see that a lot of them were insurmountable. Not only were they unavoidable, they were incapable of favorable resolution. Nonetheless, in terms of my own peace of mind and physical health, I can claim to have coped reasonably well. As a result, I have been able to meet adversity with all my resources—mental, physical, and spiritual. I could not have done so otherwise. Had I been overwhelmed by anxiety and despaired, my health would have been harmed. I would also have been constrained in my actions.

Looking around, I see that it is not only we Tibetan refugees, and members of other displaced communities, who face difficulties. Everywhere and in every society, people endure suffering and adversity—even those who enjoy freedom and material prosperity. Indeed, it seems to me that much of the unhappiness we humans endure is actually of our own making. In principle, therefore, this at least is avoidable. I also see that, in general, those individuals whose conduct is ethically positive are happier and more satisfied than those who neglect ethics. This confirms my belief that if we can reorientate our thoughts and emotions, and reorder our behavior, not only can we learn to cope with suffering more easily, but we can prevent a great deal of it from arising in the first place.

I shall try to show in this book what I mean by the term "positive ethical conduct." In doing so, I acknowledge that it is very difficult either to generalize successfully or to be absolutely precise about ethics and morality. Rarely, if ever, is any situation totally black and white. The same act will have different shades and degrees of moral value under different circumstances. At the same time, it is essential that we reach a consensus in respect to what constitutes positive conduct and what constitutes negative conduct, of what is right and what is wrong, of what is appropriate and what is inappropriate. In the past, the respect people had for religion meant that ethical practice was maintained through a majority following one religion or another. But this is no longer the case. We must therefore find some other way of establishing basic ethical principles.

Not that the reader should suppose that, as Dalai Lama, I have any special solution to offer. There is nothing in these pages which has not been said before. Indeed, I feel that the concerns and ideas expressed here are shared by many of those who think about and attempt to find solutions to the problems and suffering we humans face. In responding to the suggestion of some of my friends and offering this book to the public, my hope is to give voice to those millions who, not having an opportunity to articulate their views in public, remain members of what I take to be a silent majority.

The reader should, however, bear in mind that my formal learning has been of an entirely religious and spiritual character. Since my youth, my chief (and continuing) field of study has been Buddhist philosophy and psychology. In particular, I have studied the works of the religious philosophers of the Geluk tradition to which, by tradition, the Dalai Lamas have belonged. Being a firm believer in religious pluralism, I have also studied the principal works of other Buddhist traditions. But I have had comparatively little exposure to modern, secular thought. Yet this is not a religious book. Still less is it a book about Buddhism. My aim has been to appeal for an approach to ethics based on universal rather than religious principles.

For this reason, producing a work for a general audience has not been without challenges, and it is the result of teamwork. One particular problem arose from the fact that it is difficult to render into modern language a number of the Tibetan terms it seemed essential to use. This book is by no means intended as a philosophical treatise, so I have tried to explain these in such a way that they could be understood readily by a non-specialist readership and also rendered clearly into other languages. But in doing so, and in trying to communicate unambiguously with readers whose language and culture may be quite different from my own, it is possible that some shades of meaning in the Tibetan tongue are lost and other, unintended ones are added. I trust that careful editing has minimized this. When any such distortions come to light, I would hope to correct them in a subsequent edition. In the meantime, for his assistance in this area, for his translation into English, and for innumerable suggestions, I wish to thank Dr. Thupten Jinpa. I also wish to thank Mr. AR Norman for his work of redaction. This has been invaluable. Finally, I would like to record my thanks to those others who have helped bring this work to fruition.

—Dharamsala, February 1999

I

THE FOUNDATION
OF ETHICS

Chapter One

MODERN SOCIETY AND THE QUEST FOR HUMAN HAPPINESS

I AM A COMPARATIVE NEWCOMER TO THE modern world. Although I fled my homeland as long ago as 1959, and although my life since then as a refugee in India has brought me into much closer contact with contemporary society, my formative years were spent largely cut off from the realities of the twentieth century. This was partly due to my appointment as Dalai Lama: I became a monk at a very early age. It also reflects the fact that we Tibetans had chosen—mistakenly, in my view—to remain isolated behind the high mountain ranges which separate our country from the rest of the world.

Today, however, I travel a great deal, and it is my good fortune continuously to be meeting new people. Moreover, individuals from all walks of life come to see me. Quite a lot—especially those who make the effort to travel to the Indian hill-station at Dharamsala where I live in exile—arrive seeking something. Among these are people who have suffered greatly: some have lost parents and children; some have friends or family who committed

3

suicide; are sick with cancer and with AIDS-related illnesses. Then, of course, there are fellow Tibetans with their own tales of hardship and suffering. Unfortunately, many have unrealistic expectations, supposing that I have healing powers or that I can give some sort of blessing. But I am only an ordinary human being. The best I can do is try to help them by sharing in their suffering.

For my part, meeting innumerable others from all over the world and from every walk of life reminds me of our basic sameness as human beings. Indeed, the more I see of the world, the clearer it becomes that no matter what our situation, whether we are rich or poor, educated or not, of one race, gender, religion or another, we all desire to be happy and to avoid suffering. Our every intended action, in a sense our whole life—how we choose to live it within the context of the limitations imposed by our circumstances—can be seen as our answer to the great question which confronts us all: "How am I to be happy?"

We are sustained in this great quest for happiness, it seems to me, by hope. We know, even if we do not admit it, that there can be no guarantee of a better, happier life than the one we are leading today. As an old Tibetan proverb puts it, The next life or tomorrow—we can never be certain which will come first. But we hope to go on living. We hope that through this or that action we can bring about happiness. Everything we do, not only as individuals but also at the level of society, can be seen in terms of this fundamental aspiration. Indeed, it is one shared by all sentient beings. The desire or inclination to be happy and to avoid suffering knows no boundaries. It is in our nature. As such, it needs no justification and is validated by the simple fact that we naturally and correctly want this.

And this is precisely what we see in countries both rich and poor. Everywhere, by all means imaginable, people are striving to improve their lives. Yet strangely, my impression is that those living in the materially developed countries, for all their industry, are in some ways less satisfied, are less happy, and to some extent suffer more than those living in the least developed countries. Indeed, if we compare the rich with the poor, it often seems that those with nothing are, in fact, the least anxious, though they are plagued with physical pains and suffering. As for the rich, while a few know how to use their wealth intelligently— that is to say, not in luxurious living but by sharing it with the needy—many do not. They are so caught up with the idea of acquiring still more that they make no room for anything else in their lives. In their absorption, they actually lose the dream of happiness, which riches were to have provided. As a result, they are constantly tormented, torn between doubt about what might happen and the hope of gaining more, and plagued with mental and emotional suffering—even though outwardly they may appear to be leading entirely successful and comfortable lives. This is suggested both by the high degree and by the disturbing prevalence among the populations of the materially developed countries of anxiety, discontent, frustration, uncertainty, and depression. Moreover, this inner suffering is clearly connected with growing confusion as to what constitutes morality and what its foundations are.

I am often reminded of this paradox when I go abroad. It frequently happens that when I arrive in a new country, at first everything seems very pleasant, very beautiful. Everybody I meet is very friendly. There is nothing to complain about. But then, day by day as I listen, I hear people's problems, their concerns and worries. Below the surface, so many feel uneasy and dissatisfied with their lives. They experience feelings of isolation; then follows depression. The result is the troubled atmosphere which is such a feature of the developed world.

At first, this surprised me. Although I never imagined that material wealth alone could ever overcome suffering, looking at the developed world from Tibet, a country materially always very poor, I must admit that I thought wealth would have gone further toward reducing suffering than is actually the case. I expected that with physical hardship much reduced, as it is for the majority living in the industrially developed countries, happiness would be much easier to achieve than for those living under more severe conditions.

Instead, the extraordinary advancements of science and technology seem to have achieved little more than numerical improvement. In many cases, progress has meant hardly anything more than greater numbers of opulent houses in more cities, with more cars driving between them. Certainly there has been a reduction in some types of suffering, including especially certain illnesses. But it seems to me that there has been no overall reduction.

Saying this, I remember well an occasion on one of my early trips to the West. I was the guest of a very wealthy family who lived in a large, well-appointed house. Everyone was very charming and polite. There were servants to cater to one's every need, and I began to think that here, perhaps, was proof positive that wealth could be a source of happiness. My hosts definitely had an air of relaxed confidence. But when I saw in the bathroom, through a cupboard door which was slightly open, an array of tranquilizers and sleeping pills, I was reminded forcefully that there is often a big gap between outward appearances and inner reality.

This paradox whereby inner—or we could say psychological and emotional—suffering is so often found amid material wealth is readily apparent throughout much of the West. Indeed, it is so pervasive that we might wonder whether there is something in Western culture which predisposes people living there to such kinds of suffering? This I doubt. So many factors are involved. Clearly, material development itself has a role to play. But we can also cite the increasing urbanization of modern society, where high concentrations of people live in close proximity to one another. In this context, consider that in place of our dependence on one another for support, today, wherever possible, we tend to rely on machines and services. Whereas formerly farmers would call in all their family members to help with the harvest, today they simply telephone a contractor. We find modern living organized so that it demands the least possible direct dependence on others. The more or less universal ambition seems to be for everyone to own their own house, their own car, their own computer, and so on in order to be as independent as possible. This is natural and understandable. The increasing autonomy that people enjoy as a result of advances in science and technology has its good points. In fact, it is possible today to be far more independent of others than ever before. But with these developments, there has arisen a sense that my future is not dependent on my neighbor but rather on my job or, at most, my employer. This in turn encourages us to suppose that because others are not important for my happiness, their happiness is not important to me.

We have, in my view, created a society in which people find it harder and harder to show one another basic affection. In place of the sense of community and belonging, which we find such a reassuring feature of less wealthy (and generally rural) societies, we find a high degree of loneliness and alienation. Despite the fact that millions live in close proximity to one another, it seems that many people, especially among the old, have no one to talk to but their pets. Modern industrial society often strikes me as being like a huge self-propelled machine. Instead of human beings in charge, each individual is a tiny, insignificant component with no choice but to move when the machine moves.

All this is compounded by the contemporary rhetoric of growth and economic development which greatly reinforces people's tendency toward competitiveness and envy. And with this comes the perceived need to keep up appearances—itself a major source of problems, tension, and unhappiness. Yet the psychological and emotional suffering we find so prevalent in the West is less likely to reflect a cultural shortcoming than an underlying human tendency. Indeed, I have noticed that similar forms of inner suffering are evident outside the West. In some parts of Southeast Asia, it is observable that as prosperity has increased, traditional belief systems have begun to lose their influence over people. With this, we find a broadly similar manifestation of unease as that established in the West. This suggests that the potential exists in us all, and in the same way that physical disease reflects its environment, so it is with psychological and emotional suffering: it arises within the context of particular circumstances. Thus, in the southern, undeveloped, or "Third World" countries we find ailments broadly confined to that part of the world, such as those arising from poor sanitation. By contrast, in urban industrial societies, we see illnesses manifest in ways that are consistent with that environment. So instead of water-borne diseases, we find stress-related disease. All this implies that there are strong reasons for supposing a link between our disproportionate emphasis on external progress and the unhappiness, the anxiety, and the lack of contentment of modern society.

This may sound like a very gloomy assessment. But unless we acknowledge the extent and character of our problems, we will not be able even to begin to deal with them.

Clearly, a major reason for modern society's devotion to material progress is the very success of science and technology. Now the wonderful thing about these forms of human endeavor is that they bring immediate satisfaction. They're unlike prayer, the results of which are, for the most part, invisible—if indeed prayer works at all. And we are impressed by results. What could be more normal? Unfortunately, this devotion encourages us to suppose that the keys to happiness are material well-being on the one hand and the power conferred by knowledge on the other. And while it is obvious to anyone who gives this mature thought that the former cannot bring us happiness by itself, it is perhaps less apparent that the latter cannot. But the fact is, knowledge alone cannot provide the happiness that springs from inner

10

development, that is not reliant on external factors. Indeed, though our very detailed and specific knowledge of external phenomena is an immense achievement, the urge to reduce, to narrow down in pursuit of it, far from bringing us happiness, can actually be dangerous. It can cause us to lose touch with the wider reality of human experience and, in particular, our dependence on others.

We need also to recognize what happens when we rely too much on the external achievements of science. For example, as the influence of religion declines, there is mounting confusion with respect to the problem of how best we are to conduct ourselves in life. In the past, religion and ethics were closely intertwined. Now, many people, believing that science has "disproven" religion, make the further assumption that because there appears to be no final evidence for any spiritual authority, morality itself must be a matter of individual preference. And whereas in the past, scientists and philosophers felt a pressing need to find solid foundations on which to establish immutable laws and absolute truths, nowadays this kind of research is held to be futile. As a result, we see a complete reversal, heading toward the opposite extreme, where ultimately nothing exists any longer, where reality itself is called into question. This can only lead to chaos.

In saying this, I do not mean to criticize scientific endeavor. I have learned a great deal from my encounters with scientists, and I see no obstacle to engaging in dialogue with them even when their perspective is one of radical materialism. Indeed, for as long as I can remember, I have been fascinated by the insights of science. As a boy, there was a time when I was rather more interested in learning about the mechanics of an old film projector I found in the storerooms of the summer residence of the Dalai Lama than in my religious and scholastic studies. My concern is rather that we are apt to overlook the limitations of science. In replacing religion as the final source of knowledge in popular estimation, science begins to look a bit like another religion itself. With this comes a similar danger on the part of some of its adherents of blind faith in its principles and, correspondingly, to intolerance of alternative views. That this supplanting of religion has taken place is not surprising, however, given science's extraordinary achievements. Who could fail to be impressed at our ability to land people on the moon? Yet the fact remains that if, for example, we were to go to a nuclear physicist and say, "I am facing a moral dilemma, what should I do?" he or she could only shake their head and suggest we look elsewhere for an answer. Generally speaking, a scientist is in no better position than a lawyer in this respect. For while both science and the law can help us forecast the likely consequence of our actions, neither can tell us how we ought to act in a moral sense. Moreover, we need to recognize the limits of scientific inquiry itself. For example, though we have been aware of human consciousness for millennia, and though it has been the subject of investigation throughout history, despite scientists' best efforts they still do not understand what it actually is, nor why it exists, how it functions, nor what is its essential nature. Neither can science tell us what the substantial cause of consciousness is, nor what its effects are. Of course, consciousness belongs to that category of phenomena without form, substance, or color. It is not susceptible to investigation by external means. But this does not mean such things do not exist, merely that science cannot find them.

Should we, therefore, abandon scientific inquiry on the grounds that it has failed us? Certainly not. Nor do I mean to suggest that the goal of prosperity for all is invalid. Because of our nature, bodily and physical experience play a dominant role in our lives. The achievements of science and technology clearly reflect our desire to attain a better, more comfortable existence. This is very good. Who could fail to applaud many of the advances of modern medicine?

At the same time, I think it is genuinely true that members of certain traditional, rural communities do enjoy greater harmony and tranquility than those settled in our modern cities. For example, in the Spiti area of northern India, it remains the custom for locals not to lock their houses when they go out. It is expected that a visitor who finds the house empty would go in and help themselves to a meal while waiting for the family to return. The same obtained in Tibet in former times. This is not to say that there is no crime in such places. As in the case of pre-occupation Tibet, such things did of course happen occasionally. But when they did, people would raise their eyebrows in surprise. It was a rare and unusual event. By contrast, in some modern cities, if a day goes by without a murder, it is a remarkable event. With urbanization has come disharmony.

We must be careful not to idealize old ways of life, however. The high level of cooperation we find in undeveloped rural communities may be based more on necessity than on goodwill. People recognize it as an alternative to greater hardship. And the contentment we perceive may actually have more to do with ignorance. These people may not realize or imagine that any other way of life is possible. If they did, very likely they would embrace it eagerly. The challenge we face is therefore to find some means of enjoying the same degree of harmony and tranquility as those more traditional communities while benefiting fully from the material developments of the world as we find it at the dawn of a new millennium. To say otherwise is to imply that these communities should not even try to improve their standard of living. Yet, I am quite certain that, for example, the majority of Tibet's nomads would be very glad to have the latest thermal clothing for winter, smokeless fuel to cook with, the benefits of modern medicine, and a portable television in their tents. And I, for one, would not wish to deny them these.

Modern society, with all its benefits and defects, has emerged within the context of innumerable causes and conditions. To suppose that merely by abandoning material progress we could overcome all our problems would be shortsighted. That would be to ignore their underlying causes. Besides, there is still much in the modern world to be optimistic about.

There are countless people in the most developed countries who are active in their concern for others. Nearer home, I think of the enormous kindness we Tibetan refugees have been shown by those whose personal resources were also quite limited. For example, our children have benefited immeasurably from the selfless contribution of their Indian teachers, many of whom have been compelled to live under difficult conditions far away from their homes. On a wider scale, we might also consider the growing appreciation of fundamental human rights all over the world. This represents a very positive development in my view. The way in which the international community generally responds to natural disasters with immediate aid is also a wonderful feature of the modern world. Increasing recognition that we cannot forever continue to mistreat our natural environment without facing serious consequences is likewise a cause for hope. Moreover, I believe that, thanks largely to modern communications, people are probably more accepting of diversity now. And standards of literacy and education throughout the world are in general higher than ever before. Such positive developments I take to be an indication of what we humans are capable of.

Recently, I had the opportunity to meet the Queen Mother in England. She has been a familiar figure to me throughout my life, so this gave me great pleasure. But what was particularly encouraging was to hear her opinion, as a woman as old as the twentieth century itself, that people have become much more aware of others than when she was young. In those days, she said, people were interested mainly in their own countries whereas today there is much more concern for the inhabitants of other countries. When I asked her whether she was optimistic about the future, she replied in the affirmative without hesitation.

It is, of course, true that we can point to an abundance of severely negative trends within modern society. There is no reason to doubt the escalation in murder, violence, and rape cases year by year. In addition, we hear constantly of abusive and exploitative relationships both in the home and within the wider community, of growing numbers of young people addicted to drugs and alcohol, and of how the high proportion of marriages ending in divorce is affecting children today. Not even our own small refugee community has escaped the impact of some these developments. Whereas, for example, suicide was almost unheard of in Tibetan society, lately there have been one or two tragic incidents of this kind, even within our exile community. Likewise, whereas drug addiction among young Tibetans certainly did not exist a generation ago, we now have a few cases—mostly, it must be said, in those places where they are exposed to the modern urban lifestyle.

Yet, unlike the sufferings of sickness, old age, and death, none of these problems is by nature inevitable. Nor are they due to any lack of knowledge. When we think carefully, we see that they are all ethical problems. They each reflect our understanding of what is right and wrong, of what is positive and what is negative, of what is appropriate and what is inappropriate. But beyond this we can point to something more fundamental: a neglect of what I call our inner dimension.

What do I mean by this? According to my understanding, our overemphasis on material gain reflects an underlying assumption that what it can buy can, by itself alone, provide us with all the satisfaction we require. Yet by nature, the satisfaction material gain can provide us with will be limited to the level of the senses. If it were true that we human beings were no different from animals, this would be fine. However, given the complexity of our species—in particular, the fact of our having thoughts and emotions as well as imaginative and critical faculties—it is obvious that our needs transcend the merely sensual. The prevalence of anxiety, stress, confusion, uncertainty, and depression among those whose basic needs have been met is a clear indication of this. Our problems, both those we experience externally—such as wars, crime, and violence—and those we experience internally—our emotional and psychological sufferings—cannot be solved until we address this underlying neglect. That is why the great movements of the last hundred years and more—democracy, liberalism, socialism— have all failed to deliver the universal benefits they were supposed to provide, despite many wonderful ideas. A revolution is called for, certainly. But not a political, an economic, or even a technical revolution. We have had enough experience of these during the past century to know that a purely external approach will not suffice. What I propose is a spiritual revolution.

Chapter Two

NO MAGIC, NO MYSTERY

IN CALLING FOR A SPIRITUAL REVOLU- tion, am I advocating a religious solution to our problems after all? No. As someone nearing seventy years of age at the time of writing, I have accumulated enough experience to be completely confident that the teachings of the Buddha are both relevant and useful to humanity. If a person puts them into practice, it is certain that not only they but others, too, will benefit. My meetings with many different sorts of people the world over have, however, helped me realize that there are other faiths, and other cultures, no less capable than mine of enabling individuals to lead constructive and satisfying lives. What is more, I have come to the conclusion that whether or not a person is a religious believer does not matter much. Far more important is that they be a good human being.

I say this in acknowledgment of the fact that though a majority of the earth's nearly six billion human beings may claim allegiance to one faith tradition or another, the influence of religion on people's lives is generally marginal, especially in the developed world. It is doubtful whether globally even a billion are what I would call dedicated religious practitioners, that is to say, people who try, on a daily basis, faithfully to follow the principles and precepts of their faith. The rest remain, in this sense, non-practicing. Those who are dedicated practitioners meanwhile follow a multiplicity of religious paths. From this, it becomes clear that, given our diversity, no single religion satisfies all humanity. We may also conclude that we humans can live quite well without recourse to religious faith.

These may seem unusual statements, coming as they do from a religious figure. I am, however, Tibetan before I am Dalai Lama, and I am human before I am Tibetan. So while as Dalai Lama I have a special responsibility to Tibetans, and as a monk I have a special responsibility toward furthering interreligious harmony, as a human being I have a much larger responsibility toward the whole human family—which indeed we all have. And since the majority does not practice religion, I am concerned to try to find a way to serve all humanity without appealing to religious faith.

Actually, I believe that if we consider the world's major religions from the widest perspective, we find that they are all—Buddhism, Christianity, Hinduism, Islam, Judaism, Sikhism, Zoroastrianism, and the others—directed toward helping human beings achieve lasting happiness. And each of them is, in my opinion, capable of facilitating this. Under such circumstances, a variety of religions (each of which promotes the same basic values after all) is both desirable and useful.

Not that I always felt like this. When I was younger and living in Tibet, I believed in my heart that Buddhism was the best way. I told myself it would be marvelous if everyone converted. Yet this was due to ignorance. We Tibetans had, of course, heard of other religions. But what little we knew about them came from Tibetan translations of secondary, Buddhist sources. Naturally, these focused on those aspects of other religions which are more open to debate from a Buddhist perspective. This was not because their Bud-

20

dhist authors wished deliberately to caricature their opponents. Rather, it reflected the fact that they had no need to address all those aspects with which they had no argument since, in India, where they wrote, the works they were discussing were available in their entirety. Unfortunately, this was not the case in Tibet. There were no translations of these others scriptures available.

As I grew up, I was gradually able to learn more about the other world religions. Especially after going into exile, I began to meet people who, having dedicated their entire lives to different faiths—some through prayer and meditation, others through actively serving others—had acquired a profound experience of their particular tradition. Such personal exchanges helped me recognize the enormous value of each of the major faith traditions and led me to respect them deeply. For me, Buddhism remains the most precious path. It corresponds best with my personality. But that does not mean I believe it to be the best religion for everyone any more than I believe it necessary for everyone to be a religious believer.

Of course, both as a Tibetan and as a monk, I have been brought up according to, and educated in, the principles, the precepts, and the practice of Buddhism. I cannot, therefore, deny that my whole thinking is shaped by my understanding of what it means to be a follower of the Buddha. However, my concern in this book is to try to reach beyond the formal

boundaries of my faith. I want to show that there are indeed some universal ethical principles which could help everyone to achieve the happiness we all aspire to. Some people may feel that in this I am attempting to propagate Buddhism by stealth. But while it is difficult for me conclusively to refute the claim, this is not the case.

Actually, I believe there is an important distinction to be made between religion and spirituality. Religion I take to be concerned with faith in the claims to salvation of one faith tradition or another, an aspect of which is acceptance of some form of metaphysical or supernatural reality, including perhaps an idea of heaven or *nirvana*. Connected with this are religious teachings or dogma, ritual, prayer, and so on. Spirituality I take to be concerned with those qualities of the human spirit—such as love and compassion, patience, tolerance, forgiveness, contentment, a sense of responsibility, a sense of harmony—which bring happiness to both self and others. While ritual and prayer, along with the questions of *nirvana* and salvation, are directly connected to religious faith, these inner qualities need not be, however. There is thus no reason why the individual should not develop them, even to a high degree, without recourse to any religious or metaphysical belief system. This is why I sometimes say that religion is something we can perhaps do without. What we cannot do without are these basic spiritual qualities.

Those who practice religion would, of

course, be right to say that such qualities, or virtues, are fruits of genuine religious endeavor and that religion therefore has everything to do with developing them and with what may be called spiritual practice. But let us be clear on this point. Religious faith demands spiritual practice. Yet it seems there is much confusion, as often among religious believers or among non-believers, concerning what this actually consists in. The unifying characteristic of the qualities I have described as "spiritual" may be said to be some level of concern for others' well-being. In Tibetan, we speak of *shen pen kyi sem* meaning "the thought to be of help to others." And when we think about them, we see that each of the qualities noted is defined by an implicit concern for others' well-being. Moreover, the one who is compassionate, loving, patient, tolerant, forgiving, and so on to some extent recognizes the potential impact of their actions on others and orders their conduct accordingly. Thus spiritual practice according to this description involves, on the one hand, acting out of concern for others' well-being. On the other, it entails transforming ourselves so that we become more readily disposed to do so. To speak of spiritual practice in any terms other than these is meaningless.

My call for a spiritual revolution is thus not a call for a religious revolution. Nor is it a reference to a way of life that is somehow otherworldly, still less to something magical or mysterious. Rather, it is a call for a radical reorientation away from our habitual preoccupation with self. It is a call to turn toward the wider community of beings with whom we are connected, and for conduct which recognizes others' interests alongside our own.

Here the reader may object that while the transformation of character that such a reorientation implies is certainly desirable, and while it is good that people develop compassion and love, a revolution of spirit is hardly adequate to solve the variety and magnitude of problems we face in the modern world. Furthermore, it could be argued that problems arising from, for example, violence in the home, addiction to drugs and alcohol, family breakup, and so on are better understood and tackled on their own terms. Nevertheless, given that they could each certainly be solved through people being more loving and compassionate toward one another—however improbable this may seem—they can also be characterized as spiritual problems susceptible to a spiritual solution. This is not to say that all we need do is cultivate spiritual values and these problems will automatically disappear. On the contrary, each of them needs a specific solution. But we find that when this spiritual dimension is neglected, we have no hope of achieving a lasting solution.

Why is this? Bad news is a fact of life. Each time we pick up a newspaper, or turn on the television or radio, we are confronted with sad tidings. Not a day goes by but, somewhere in the world, something happens that everyone agrees is unfortunate. No matter where we are from or what our philosophy of life, to a greater or lesser extent, we are all sorry to hear of others' suffering.

These events can be divided into two broad categories: those which have principally natural causes—earthquakes, drought, floods, and the like—and those which are of human origin. Wars, crime, violence of every sort, corruption, poverty, deception, fraud, and social, political, and economic injustice are each the consequence of negative human behavior. And who is responsible for such behavior? We are. From royalty, presidents, prime ministers, and politicians through administrators, scientists, doctors, lawyers, academics, students, priests, nuns and monks, such as myself, to industrialists, artists, shopkeepers, technicians, pieceworkers, manual laborers, and those without work, there is not a single class or sector of society which does not contribute to our daily diet of unhappy news.

Fortunately, unlike natural disasters, which we can do little or nothing about, these human problems, because they are all essentially ethical problems, can be overcome. The fact that there are so many people, again from every sector and level of society, working to do so is a reflection of this intuition: There are those who join political parties to fight for a fairer constitution; those who become lawyers to fight for justice; those who join aid organizations to fight poverty; those who care, both on a professional and on a voluntary basis, for the victims of harm. Indeed, we are all, according to our own understanding and in our own way, trying to make the world—or at least our bit of it—a better place for us to live in.

Unfortunately, we find that no matter how sophisticated and well administered our legal systems, and no matter how advanced our methods of external control, by themselves these cannot eradicate wrongdoing. Observe that nowadays our police forces have at their disposal technology that could barely have been imagined fifty years ago. They have methods of surveillance which enable them to see what formerly was hidden; they have DNA matching, forensic laboratories, sniffer dogs, and, of course, highly trained personnel. Yet criminal methods are correspondingly advanced so that really we are no better off. Where ethical restraint is lacking, there can be no hope of overcoming problems like those of rising crime. In fact, without such inner discipline, we find that the very means we use to solve them becomes a source of difficulty itself. The increasing sophistication of criminal and police methods is a vicious and mutually reinforcing cycle.

What, then, is the relationship between spirituality and ethical practice? Since love and compassion and similar qualities all, by definition, presume some level of concern for others' well-being, they presume ethical restraint. We cannot be loving and compassionate unless at the same time we curb our own harmful impulses and desires.

As to the foundations of ethical practice itself, it might be supposed that here at least I advocate a religious approach. Certainly, each of the major religious traditions has a well-developed ethical system. However, the difficulty with tying our understanding of right and wrong to religion is that we must then ask, "Which religion?" Which articulates the most complete, the most accessible, the most acceptable system? The arguments would never stop. Moreover, to do so would be to ignore the fact that many who reject religion do so out of convictions sincerely held, not merely because they are unconcerned with the deeper questions of human existence. We cannot suppose that such people are without a sense of right and wrong or of what is morally appropriate just because some who are anti-religion are immoral. Besides, religious belief is no guarantee of moral integrity. Looking at the history of our species, we see that among the major troublemakers—those who visited violence, brutality, and destruction on their fellow human beings—there have been many who professed religious faith, often loudly. Religion can help us establish basic ethical principles. Yet we can still talk about ethics and morality without having recourse to religion.

Again, it could be objected that if we do not accept religion as the source of ethics, we must allow that people's understanding of what is good and right, of what is wrong and bad, of what is morally appropriate and what is not, of what constitutes a positive act and what a negative act must vary according to circumstances and even from person to person. But here let me say that no one should suppose it could ever be possible to devise a set of rules or laws to provide us with the answer to every ethical dilemma, even if we were to accept religion as the basis of morality. Such a formulaic approach could never hope to capture the richness and diversity of human experience. It would also give grounds for arguing that we are responsible only to the letter of those laws, rather than for our actions.

This is not to say that it is useless to attempt to construe principles which can be understood as morally binding. On the contrary, if we are to have any hope of solving our problems, it is essential that we find a way to do so. We must have some means of adjudicating between, for example, terrorism as a means to political reform and Mahatma Gandhi's principles of peaceful resistance. We must be able to show that violence toward others is wrong. And yet we must find some way of doing so which avoids the extremes of crude absolutism on the one hand, and of trivial relativism on the other.

My own view, which does not rely solely on religious faith or even on an original idea, but rather on ordinary common sense, is that establishing binding ethical principles is possible when we take as our starting point the observation that we all desire happiness and wish to avoid suffering. We have no means of discriminating between right and wrong if we do not take into account others' feelings, others' suffering. For this reason, and also because—as we shall see—the notion of absolute truth is difficult to sustain outside the context of religion, ethical conduct is not something we engage in because it is somehow right in itself but because, like ourselves, all others desire to be happy and to avoid suffering. Given that this is a natural disposition, shared by all, it follows that each individual has a right to pursue this goal. Accordingly, I suggest that one of the things which determines whether an act is ethical or not is its effect on others' experience or expectation of happiness. An act which harms or does violence to this is potentially an unethical act.

I say *potentially* because although the consequences of our actions are important, there are other factors to consider, including both the question of intent and the nature of the act itself. We can all think of things which we have done that have upset others, despite the fact that it was by no means our intention to do so. Similarly, it is also not hard to think of acts which, though they may appear somewhat forceful and aggressive and likely to cause hurt, could yet contribute to others' happiness in the long run. Disciplining children will often fall into this category. On the other hand, the fact that our actions may appear to be gentle does not mean that they are positive or ethical if our intentions are selfish. On the contrary, if, for example, our intention is to mislead, then to pretend kindness is a most unfortunate deed. Though force may not be involved, such an act is certainly violent. It does violence not only insofar as the end is harmful to the other but also in that it injures that person's trust and expectation of truth.

Again, it is not difficult to imagine a case where an individual may suppose their actions to be well intended and directed toward the greater good of others, but where they are in reality totally immoral. Here we might think of a soldier who carries out orders summarily to execute civilian prisoners. Believing the cause to be a just one, this soldier may suppose such actions are directed toward the greater good of humanity. Yet, according to the principle of non-violence I have put forward, such killing would by definition be an unethical act. Carrying out these orders would thus be gravely negative conduct. In other words, the content of our actions is also important in determining whether they are ethical or not, since certain acts are negative by definition.

The factor which is perhaps most important of all in determining the ethical nature of an act is neither its content nor its consequence, however. In fact, since only rarely are the fruits of our actions directly attributable to us alone—whether the helmsman is able to bring his boat to safety in a storm depends not just on his actions—consequence could conceivably be the least important factor. In Tibetan, the term for what is considered to be of the greatest significance in determining the ethical value of a given action is the individual's *kun long*. Translated literally, the participle *kun* means "thoroughly" or "from the depths," and "long (wa)" denotes the act of causing something to stand up, to arise, or to awaken. But in the sense in which it used here, *kun long* is understood as that which drives or inspires our actions—both those we intend directly and those which are in a sense involuntary. It therefore denotes the individual's overall state of heart and mind. When this is wholesome, it follows that our actions themselves will be (ethically) wholesome.

From this description, it is clear that it is difficult to translate *kun long* succinctly. Generally, it is rendered simply as "motivation," but this clearly does not capture the full range of its meaning. The word "disposition," although it comes quite close, lacks the active sense of the Tibetan. On the other hand, to use the phrase "overall state of heart and mind" seems unnecessarily long. Arguably, it could be abbreviated to "mind-state," but this would ignore the wider meaning of mind as it is used in Tibetan. The word for "mind," *lo,* includes the ideas of consciousness, or awareness, alongside those of feeling and emotion. This reflects an understanding that emotions and thoughts cannot ultimately be separated. Even the perception of a quality, like color, is held to carry within it an affective dimension. Nor is there an idea of pure sensation without any accompanying cognitive event. The inference is rather that we can identify different types of emotion. There are those which are primarily instinctual, such as revulsion at the sight of blood, and there are those which have a more developed rational component, such as fear of poverty. The reader is asked to remember this point whenever I speak of "mind," of "motivation," of "disposition," or of "states of mind."

That this is so, that the individual's overall state of heart and mind, or motivation, in the moment of action is, generally speaking, the key to determining its ethical content, is easily understood when we consider how our actions are affected when we are gripped with powerful negative thoughts and emotions such as hatred and anger. In that moment, our mind and heart (*lo*) are in turmoil. Not only does this cause us to lose our sense of proportion and perspective, but we also lose sight of the likely impact of our actions on others. Indeed, we can become so distracted that we ignore the question of others, and of their right to happiness, altogether. Our actions under such circumstances—that is to say our deeds, words, thoughts, omissions, and desires—will almost certainly be injurious of others' happiness. And this in spite of what our long-term intentions toward others may be or whether our actions are consciously intended or not. Consider a situation where we become embroiled in an argument with a family member. How we deal with the charged atmosphere which develops will depend to a large extent on what underlies our actions at that moment—in other words, our *kun long*. The less calm we are, the more likely we are to react negatively with harsh words, and the more certain we are to say or do things which later we regret bitterly, even though we feel deeply for that person.

Or imagine a situation where we inconvenience another in some small way, perhaps by bumping into them accidentally while walking along, and they shout at us for being careless. We are much more likely to shrug this off if our disposition (*kun long*) is wholesome, if our hearts are suffused with compassion, than if we are under the sway of negative emotions. When the driving force of our actions is wholesome, our actions will tend automatically to contribute to others' well-being. They will thus automatically be ethical. Further, the more this is our habitual state, the less likely we are to react badly when provoked. And even when we do lose our temper, any outburst will be free of any sense of malice or hatred. The aim of spiritual and, therefore, ethical practice is thus to transform and perfect the individual's *kun long*. This is how we become better human beings.

We find that the more we succeed in transforming our hearts and minds through cultivating spiritual qualities, the better able we will be to cope with adversity and the greater the likelihood that our actions will be ethically wholesome. So if I may be permitted to give my own case as an example, this understanding of ethics means that in striving continuously to cultivate a positive, or wholesome, mind-state I try to be of the greatest service to others that I can be. By making sure, in addition to this, that the content of my actions is, so far as I am able to make them, similarly positive, I reduce my chances of acting unethically. How effective this strategy is, that is to say, what the consequences are in terms of others' well-being, either in the short-term or the long-term, there is no way to tell. But, provided my efforts are continual and provided I pay attention, no matter what happens, I should never have cause for regret. At least I know I have done my best.

My description in this chapter of the relationship between ethics and spirituality does not address the question of how we are to resolve ethical dilemmas. We will come to that later. Rather, I have been concerned to outline an approach to ethics which, by relating ethical discourse to the basic human experience of happiness and suffering, avoids the problems which arise when we ground ethics in religion. The reality is that the majority of people today are unpersuaded of the need for religion. Moreover, there may be conduct which is acceptable to one religious tradition but not to another. As to what I meant by the term "spiritual revolution," I trust that I have made it clear that a spiritual revolution entails an ethical revolution.

Chapter Three

DEPENDENT ORIGINATION AND THE NATURE OF REALITY

AT A PUBLIC TALK I GAVE IN JAPAN A FEW years ago, I saw some people coming toward me carrying a bunch of flowers. I stood up in anticipation of receiving their offering, but to my surprise, they walked straight past and laid the flowers on the altar behind me. I sat down feeling somewhat embarrassed! Yet again I was reminded that the way in which things and events unfold does not always coincide with our expectations. Indeed, this fact of life—that there is often a gap between the way in which we perceive phenomena and the reality of a given situation—is the source of much unhappiness. This is especially true when, as in the example here, we make judgments on the basis of a partial understanding, which turns out not to be fully justified.

Before considering what a spiritual and ethical revolution might consist in, let us therefore give some thought to the nature of reality itself. The close connection between how we perceive ourselves in relation to the world we inhabit and our behavior in response to it means that our understanding of phenomena is crucially significant. If we don't understand phenomena, we are more likely to do things to harm ourselves and others.

When we consider the matter, we start to see that we cannot finally separate out any phenomena from the context of other phenomena. We can only really speak in terms of relationships. In the course of our daily lives, we engage in countless different activities and receive huge sensory input from all that we encounter. The problem of misperception, which, of course, varies in degree, usually arises because of our tendency to isolate particular aspects of an event or experience and see them as constituting its totality. This leads to a narrowing of perspective and from there to false expectations. But when we consider reality itself we quickly become aware of its infinite complexity, and we realize that our habitual perception of it is often inadequate. If this were not so, the concept of deception would be meaningless. If things and events always unfolded as we expected, we would have no notion of illusion or of misconception.

As a means to understanding this complexity, I find the concept of dependent origination (in Tibetan, *ten del*), articulated by the Madhyamika (Middle Way) school of Buddhist philosophy, to be particularly helpful. According to this, we can understand how things and events come to be in three different ways. At the first level, the principle of cause and effect, whereby all things and events arise in dependence on a complex web of interrelated causes and conditions, is invoked. This suggests that no thing or event can be construed as capable of coming into, or remaining in, existence by itself. For example, if I take some clay and mold it, I can bring a pot into being. The pot exists as an effect of my actions. At the same time, it is also the effect of a myriad of other causes and conditions. These include the combination of clay and water to form its raw material. Beyond this, we can point to the coming together of the molecules, the atoms, and other minute particles which form these constituents (which are themselves dependent on innumerable other factors). Then there are the circumstances leading up to my decision to make a pot. And there are the co-operative conditions of my actions as I give shape to the clay. All these different factors make it clear that my pot cannot come into existence independently of its causes and conditions. Rather it is dependently originated.

On the second level, *ten del* can be understood in terms of the mutual dependence which exists between parts and whole. Without parts, there can be no whole; without a whole, the concept of parts makes no sense. The idea of "whole" is predicated on parts, but these parts themselves must be considered to be wholes comprised of their own parts.

On the third level, all phenomena can be understood to be dependently originated because, when we analyze them, we find that, ultimately, they lack independent identity. This can be understood from the way in which we refer to certain phenomena. For example, the words "action" and "agent" presuppose one another. So do "parent" and "child." Someone is a parent only because he or she has children. Likewise, a daughter or son is so called only in relation to them having parents. The same relationship of mutual dependence is seen in the language we use to describe trades or professions. Individuals are called farmers on account of their work on the land. Doctors are so called because of their work in field of medicine.

In a more subtle way, things and events can be understood in terms of dependent origination when, for example, we ask, What exactly is a clay pot? When we look for something we can describe as its final identity, we find that the pot's very existence—and by implication that of all other phenomena—is to some extent provisional and determined by convention. When we ask whether its identity is determined by its shape, its function, its specific parts (that is, its being compounded of clay, water, and so on), we find that the term "pot" is merely a verbal designation. There is no single characteristic which can be said to identify it. Nor indeed does the totality of its characteristics. We can imagine pots of different shapes that are no less pots. And because we can only really speak of its existing in relation to a complex nexus of causes and conditions, viewed from this perspective, it has no one defining quality. In other words, it does not exist in and of itself, but rather it is dependently originated.

As far as mental phenomena are concerned, we see that again there is a dependence. Here it lies between perceiver and perceived. Take, for example, the perception of a flower. First, in order for such a perception to arise, there must be a sense organ. Second, there must be a condition—in this case the flower itself. Third, in order for a perception to occur, there must be something which directs the focus of the perceiver to the object. Then, through the causal interaction of these conditions, a cognitive event occurs which we call the perception of a flower. Now let us examine what exactly constitutes this event. Is it only the operation of the sense faculty? Is it only the interaction between that faculty and the flower itself? Or is it something else? We find that in the end, we cannot understand the concept of perception except in the context of an indefinitely complex series of causes and conditions.

If we take consciousness itself as the object of our investigation, although we tend to think of it in terms of something intrinsic and unchangeable, we find that it, too, is better understood in terms of dependent origination. This is because apart from individual perceptual, cognitive, and emotional experiences, it is difficult to posit an independently existing entity. Rather, consciousness is more like a construct which arises out of a spectrum of complex events.

Another way to understand the concept of dependent origination is to consider the phenomena of time. Ordinarily, we suppose that there is an independently existing entity which we call time. We speak of time past, present, and future. However, when we look more closely, we see that again this concept is merely a convention. We find that the term "present moment" is just a label denoting the interface between the tenses "past" and "future." We cannot actually pinpoint the present. Just a fraction of a second before the supposed present moment lies the past; just a fraction of a second after it lies the future. Yet if we say that the present moment is "now," no sooner have we spoken the word than it lies in the past. If we were to maintain that nevertheless there must be a single moment which is indivisible into either past or future, we would, in fact, have no grounds for any separation into past, present, and future at all. If there is a single moment which is indivisible, then we would have only the present. But without a concept of the present, it becomes difficult to speak about the past and the future since both clearly depend on the present. Moreover, if we were to conclude from our analysis that the present does not then exist, we would have to deny not only worldly convention but also our own experience. Indeed, when we begin to analyze our experience of time, we find that here the past disappears and the future is yet to come. We experience only the present.

Where do these observations leave us? Certainly, things become somewhat more complex when we think along these lines. The more satisfactory conclusion is surely to say that the present does indeed exist. But we cannot conceive of it doing so inherently or objectively. The present comes into being in dependence on the past and the future.

How does this help us? What is the value of these observations? They have a number of important implications. Firstly, when we come to see that everything we perceive and experience arises as a result of an indefinite series of interrelated causes and conditions, our whole perspective changes. We begin to see that the universe we inhabit can be understood in terms of a living organism where each cell works in balanced cooperation with every other cell to sustain the whole. If, then, just one of these cells is harmed, as when disease strikes, that balance is harmed and there is danger to the whole. This, in turn, suggests that our individual well-being is intimately connected both with that of all others and with the environment within which we live. It also becomes apparent that our every action, our every deed, word, and thought, no matter how slight or inconsequential it may seem, has an implication not only for ourselves but for all others, too.

Furthermore, when we view reality in terms of dependent origination, it draws us away from our usual tendency to see things and events in terms of solid, independent, discrete entities. This is helpful because it is this tendency which causes us to exaggerate one or two aspects of our experience and make them representative of the whole reality of a given situation while ignoring its wider complexities.

Such an understanding of reality as suggested by this concept of dependent origination also presents us with a significant challenge. It challenges us to see things and events less in terms of black and white and more in terms of a complex interlinking of relationships, which are hard to pin down. And it makes it difficult to speak in terms of absolutes. Moreover, if all phenomena are dependent on other phenomena, and if no phenomena can exist independently, even our most cherished selves must be considered not to exist in the way we normally assume. Indeed, we find that if we search for the identity of the self analytically, its apparent solidity dissolves even more readily than that of the clay pot or that of the present moment. For whereas a pot is something concrete we can actually point to, the self is more elusive: its identity as a construct quickly becomes evident. We come to see that the habitual sharp distinction we make between "self" and "others" is to some extent an exaggeration.

This is not to deny that every human being naturally and correctly has a strong sense of "I." Even though we might not be able to say why it is so, this sense of self is certainly there. But let us examine what constitutes the actual object we call self. Is it the mind? Sometimes it happens that an individual's mind becomes hyperactive, or it may become depressed. In either case, a doctor may prescribe medicine in order to improve that person's sense of well-being. This shows that generally we think of the mind as the possession of the self. And, indeed, when we think closely, statements such as "my body," "my speech," "my mind" all have within them an implied notion of ownership. It is difficult, therefore, to see how mind can constitute self, although it is true that there have been Buddhist philosophers who tried to identify self with consciousness. Were self and consciousness the same thing, it would follow, absurdly, that the actor and the action, both the doer and what is done of knowing, are one and the same. We would have to say that the agent "I" who knows and the process of knowing are identical. On this view, it is also hard to see how the self could exist as an independent phenomenon outside the mind-body aggregate. This suggests that the word "self" does not denote an independent object. Rather it is a label for a complex web of interrelated phenomena.

Here let us step back and review how we normally relate to this idea of self. We say, "I am tall; I am short; I did this; I did that," and nobody questions us. It is quite clear what we mean, and everybody is happy to accept the convention. On this level, we exist quite in accordance with these statements. Such convention is part of everyday discourse and is compatible with common experience. But this does not mean that something exists solely because it is said to or because there is a word that refers to it. No one has ever found a unicorn.

Conventions may be said to be valid when they do not contradict knowledge acquired either through empirical experience or through inference, and when they serve as the foundation for a common discourse within which we situate such notions as truth and falsity. This does not preclude us from accepting that, although perfectly adequate as a convention, the self, as with all other phenomena, exists in dependence on the labels and concepts we apply to the term. Consider in this context an instance where, in the dark, we mistake a coiled rope for a snake. We stop still and feel afraid. Although what we see is in reality a length of rope we have forgotten about, because of the lack of light and due to our misconception, we think it is a snake. Actually, the coil of rope possesses not the slightest property of a snake other than in the way it appears to us. The snake itself is not there. We have imputed its existence onto an inanimate object. So it is with the notion of an independently existing self.

We also find that the very concept of self is relative. Here consider the fact that we often find ourselves in situations where we blame ourselves. We say, "Oh, on such and such a day I really let myself down," and we speak of feeling angry with ourselves. This would suggest that there are in fact two distinct selves, the one which did wrong and the one which criticizes. The former is a self understood in relation to a particular experience or event. The latter is understood from a perspective of the self as a generality. Yet even though it makes sense to have an internal dialogue like this, still there is only one continuum of consciousness at any given moment. Similarly, we can see that the personal identity of a single individual has many different aspects. In my own case, for example, there is a perception of a self that is a monk, of a self that is Tibetan, of a self that is from the Amdo region of Tibet, and so on. Some of these selves predate others. For instance, the "self" which is Tibetan existed before the "self" that is a monk. I did not become a novice monk until I was seven years old. The "self" which is a refugee has only existed since 1959. In other words, on one single basis there are many designations. They are all Tibetan since that "self"—or identity—existed at my birth. But they are all nominally different. To me, this is further reason to have doubts about the inherent existence of self. We cannot, therefore, say that any one characteristic is what finally constitutes my self or, on the other hand, is the sum of them. For even if I were to relinquish one or more, the sense of "I" would still continue.

There is thus no single thing that can be found under analysis to identify the self. Just as when we try to find the ultimate identity of a solid object, it eludes us. Indeed, we are forced to conclude that this precious thing which we take such care of, which we go to such lengths to protect and make comfortable, is, in the end, no more substantial than a rainbow in the summer sky.

If it is true that no object or phenomena, not even the self, exists inherently, should we then conclude that, ultimately, nothing exists at all? Or is the reality we perceive simply a projection of the mind, apart from which nothing exists? No. When we say that things and events can only be established in terms of their dependently originating nature, that they are without intrinsic reality, existence, or identity, we are not denying the existence of phenomena altogether. The "identityless-ness" of phenomena points rather to the way in which things exist: not independently but in a sense interdependently. Far from under-mining the notion of phenomenal reality, I believe the concept of dependent origination provides a robust framework within which to situate cause and effect, truth and falsity, identity and difference, harm and benefit. It is, therefore, quite wrong to infer from the idea any sort of nihilistic approach to reality. A simple nothingness, without any sense of an object being this and not that, is absolutely not my meaning. Indeed if we take lack of intrinsic identity as the object of further inquiry and search for its true nature, what we find is the identitylessness of identitylessness and so on, going into infinity—from which we must conclude that even the absence of intrinsic exis-tence exists only conventionally. So while acknowledging that there is often a discrepancy between perception and reality, it is important not to go to the extreme of supposing that behind the phenomenal is a realm which is somehow more "real." The problem with this is that we may then dismiss everyday experience as nothing but an illusion. That would be quite wrong.

One of the most promising developments in modern science is the emergence of quantum and probability theory. To some degree at least, this appears to support the notion of the dependent origination of phenomena. Although I cannot claim to have a very clear understanding of this theory, the observation that at the subatomic level it becomes difficult to distinguish clearly between the observer of an object and the object itself seems to indicate a movement toward the conception of reality I have outlined. I would not wish to emphasize this too strongly, however. What science holds to be true today is liable to change. New discoveries mean that what is accepted today may be doubted tomorrow. Besides, on whatever premise we base our appreciation of the fact that things and events do not exist independently, the consequences are similar.

Such an understanding of reality allows us to see that the sharp distinction we make between self and others arises largely as a result of conditioning. Yet it is possible to imagine becoming habituated to an extended conception of self wherein the individual situates his or her interests within that of others' interests. For example, when an individual thinks in terms of his or her homeland, and says, "We are Tibetan" or "We are French," they understand their identity in terms of something that goes beyond that of the individual self.

If the self had intrinsic identity, it would be possible to speak in terms of self-interest in isolation from that of others'. But because this is not so, because self and others can only really be understood in terms of relationship, we see that self-interest and others' interest are closely interrelated. Indeed, within this picture of dependently originated reality, we see that there is no self-interest completely unrelated to others' interests. Due to the fundamental interconnectedness which lies at the heart of reality, your interest is also my interest. From this, it becomes clear that "my" interest and "your" interest are intimately connected. In a deep sense, they converge.

Accepting a more complex understanding of reality where all things and events are seen to be closely interrelated does not mean we cannot infer that the ethical principles we identified earlier cannot be understood as binding, even if, on this view, it becomes difficult to speak in terms of absolutes, at least outside a religious context. On the contrary, the concept of dependent origination compels us to take the reality of cause and effect with utmost seriousness. By this I mean the fact that particular causes lead to particular effects, and that certain actions lead to suffering while others lead to happiness. It is in everybody's interest to do what leads to happiness and avoid that which leads to suffering. And because, as we have seen, our interests are inextricably linked, we are compelled to accept ethics as the indispensable interface between my desire to be happy and yours.

Chapter Four

REDEFINING THE GOAL

I HAVE OBSERVED THAT WE ALL NATUrally desire happiness and not to suffer. I have suggested, furthermore, that these are rights, from which in my opinion we can infer that an ethical act is one which does not harm others' experience or expectation of happiness. And I have described an understanding of reality which points to a commonality of interest in respect to self and others.

Let us now consider the nature of happiness. The first thing to note is that it is a relative quality. We experience it differently according to our circumstances. What makes one person glad may be a source of suffering to another. Most of us would be extremely sorry to be sent to prison for life. Yet a criminal under threat of the death penalty would likely be very happy to be reprieved with a sentence of life imprisonment. Second, it is important to recognize that we use the same word "happiness" to describe very different states, although this is more obvious in Tibetan where the same word, *de wa,* is also used for "pleasure." We speak of happiness in connection with bathing in cool water on a hot day. We speak of it in connection with certain ideal states, such as when we say, "I would be so happy to win the lottery." We also speak of happiness in relation to the simple joys of family life.

In this last case, happiness is more of a state that persists in spite of ups and downs and occasional intermissions. But in the case of bathing in cool water on a hot day, because it is the consequence of an activity which seeks to please the senses, it is necessarily transient. If we remain in the water too long, we start to feel cold. Indeed, the happiness we derive from such activities depends on their being short-lived. In the case of winning a large sum of money, the question of whether it would confer lasting happiness or merely the sort that is soon overwhelmed by problems and difficulties that cannot be solved by wealth alone depends on the one who wins it. But generally speaking, even if money brings us happiness, it tends to be of the kind which money can buy: material things and sensory experiences. And these, we discover, become a source of suffering themselves. So far as actual possessions are concerned, for example, we must admit that often they cause us more, not less, difficulties in life. The car breaks down, we lose our money, our most precious belongings are stolen, our house is damaged by fire. Either that or we suffer because we worry about these things happening.

If this were not the case—if in fact such actions and circumstances did not contain within them the seed of suffering—the more we indulged in them, the greater our happiness would be, just as pain increases the more we endure the causes of pain. But such is not the case. In fact, while occasionally we may feel we have found perfect happiness of this sort, this seeming perfection turns out to be as ephemeral as a drop of dew on a leaf, shining brilliantly one moment, gone the next.

This explains why placing too much hope in material development is a mistake. The problem is not materialism as such. Rather it is the underlying assumption that full satisfaction can arise from gratifying the senses alone. Unlike animals, whose quest for happiness is restricted to survival and to the immediate gratification of sensory desires, we human beings have the capacity to experience happiness at a deeper level, which, when achieved, has the capacity to overwhelm contrary experiences. Consider the case of a soldier who fights in a battle. He is wounded, but the battle is won. The satisfaction he experiences in victory means that his experience of suffering on account of his wounds will likely be far less than that of a soldier with the same wounds on the losing side.

This human capacity for experiencing deeper levels of happiness also explains why such things as music and the arts offer a greater degree of happiness and satisfaction than merely acquiring material objects. However, even though aesthetic experiences are a source of happiness, they still have a strong sensory component. Music depends on the ears, art on the eyes, dance on the body. As with the satisfactions we derive from work or career, they are in general acquired through the senses. By themselves, these cannot offer the happiness we dream of.

Now, it could be argued that while it is all very well to distinguish happiness that is transient from that which is lasting, between ephemeral and genuine happiness, the only happiness it is meaningful to speak of when a person is dying from thirst is access to water. This is unarguable. When it comes to the question of survival, naturally our needs become so urgent that the majority of our effort will go toward fulfilling them. Yet because the urge to survival comes out of physical need, it follows that bodily satisfaction is invariably limited to what the senses can provide. So to conclude that we should seek immediate gratification of the senses in all circumstances would hardly be justified. Actually, when we think carefully, we see that the brief elation we experience when appeasing sensual impulses may not be very different from what the drug addict feels when indulging his or her habit. Temporary relief is soon followed by a craving for more. And in just the same way that taking drugs in the end only causes trouble, so, too, does much of what we undertake to fulfill our immediate sensory desires. This is not to say that the pleasure we take in certain activities is somehow mistaken. But we must acknowledge that there can be no hope of gratifying the senses permanently. At best, the happiness we derive from eating a good meal can only last until the next time we are hungry. As one ancient Indian writer remarked: *Indulging our senses and drinking salt water are alike: the more we partake, the more our desire and thirst grow.*

Indeed, we find that a great deal of what I have called internal suffering can be attributed to our impulsive approach to happiness. We do not stop to consider the complexity of a given situation. Our tendency is to rush in and do what seems to promise the shortest route to satisfaction. But in doing so, all too frequently we deprive ourselves of the opportunity for a greater degree of fulfillment. This is actually quite strange. Usually we do not allow our children to do whatever they want. We realize that if given their freedom, they would probably spend their time playing rather than studying. So instead we make them sacrifice the immediate pleasure of play and compel them to study. Our strategy is more long term. And while this may be less fun for them, it confers a solid foundation for their future. But as adults, we often neglect this principle. We overlook the fact that if, for example, one partner in a marriage devotes all their time to their own narrow interests, it is sure that the other partner will suffer. And when that happens, it is inevitable the marriage will become harder and harder to sustain. Similarly, we fail to recognize that when the parents are interested only in each other and neglect their children, there are sure to be negative consequences.

When we act to fulfill our immediate desires without taking into account others' interests, we undermine the possibility of lasting happiness. Consider that if we live in a neighborhood with ten other families and yet we never give a thought to their well-being, we rob ourselves of the opportunity to benefit from their society. On the other hand, if we make the effort to be friendly and have regard for their well-being, we provide for our own happiness as well as theirs. Or again, imagine an instance where we meet somebody new. Perhaps we go for a meal together. Now this may cost us some money. But as a result, there is a good chance of founding a relationship, which brings many benefits over the years to come. Conversely, if on meeting someone we see a chance to defraud them, and we take it, though we have gained a sum of money instantly, the likelihood is that we have completely destroyed the possibility of a long-term benefit from interaction with them.

Let us now consider the nature of what I have

characterized as genuine happiness. Here my own experience might serve to illustrate the state to which I refer. As a Buddhist monk, I have been trained in the practice, the philosophy, and the principles of Buddhism. But as to any sort of practical education to cope with the demands of modern living, I have received almost none. During the course of my life, I have had to handle enormous responsibilities and difficulties. At sixteen, I lost my freedom when Tibet was occupied. At twenty-four, I lost my country itself when I came into exile. For forty years now I have lived as a refugee in a foreign country, albeit the one that it is my spiritual home. Throughout this time, I have been trying to serve my fellow refugees and, to the extent possible, the Tibetans who remain in Tibet. Meanwhile, our homeland has known immeasurable destruction and suffering. And, of course, I have lost not only my mother and other close family members but also dear friends. Yet for all this, although I certainly feel sad when I think about these losses, still so far as my basic serenity is concerned, on most days I am calm and contented. Even when difficulties arise, as they must, I am usually not much bothered by them. I have no hesitation in saying that I am happy.

According to my experience, the principal characteristic of genuine happiness is peace: inner peace. By this I do not mean some kind of feeling of being "spaced out." Nor am I speaking of an absence of feeling. On the contrary, the peace I am describing is rooted in concern for others and involves a high degree of sensitivity and feeling, although I cannot claim personally to have succeeded very far in this. Rather, I attribute my sense of peace to the effort to develop concern for others.

This fact, that inner peace is the principal characteristic of happiness, explains the paradox that while we can all think of people who remain dissatisfied, despite having every material advantage, there are others who remain happy, notwithstanding the most difficult circumstances. Consider the example of those eighty thousand Tibetans who, during the months following my escape into exile, left Tibet for the sanctuary offered them by the Indian government. The conditions they faced were hard in the extreme. There was little food available and even less medicine. The refugee camps could offer no better accommodation than canvas tents. Most people had few possessions beyond the clothes they had left home in. They wore heavy *chubas* (the traditional Tibetan dress) appropriate to our harsh winters, when what they really needed in India was the lightest cotton. And there was terrible sickness from diseases unknown in Tibet. Yet for all their hardship, today the survivors exhibit few signs of trauma. Even then, few entirely lost confidence. Fewer still gave in to their feelings of sorrow and despair. I would even say that once the initial shock had passed, the majority remained quite optimistic and, yes, happy.

The indication here is that if we can develop this quality of inner peace, no matter what difficulties we meet with in life, our basic sense of well-being will not be undermined. It also follows that though there is no denying the importance of external factors in bringing this about, we are mistaken if we suppose that they can ever make us completely happy.

Certainly our constitution, our upbringing, and our circumstances all contribute to our experience of happiness. And we can all agree that the lack of certain things makes its attainment all the harder. So let us consider these in turn. Good health, friends, freedom, and a degree of prosperity are all valuable and helpful. Good health speaks for itself. We all desire it. Similarly, we all need and want friends, no matter what our situation or how successful we become. I have always been fascinated by watches, but although I am particularly fond of the one I generally wear, it never shows me any affection. In order to attain the satisfaction of love, we need friends who can return our affection. Of course, there are different kinds of friends. There are those who are really the friend of status, money, and fame, and not friends of the person who possess these things. But I refer to those who are there to help us when we encounter a difficult stage in life and not those who base their relationship with us on superficial attributes.

Freedom, in the sense of liberty to pursue happiness and to hold and express personal views, likewise contributes to our sense of inner peace. In societies where this is not permitted, we find spies who pry into the lives of every community, even the family itself. The inevitable result is that people start to lose confidence in one another. They become suspicious and doubt others' motives. Once a person's basic sense of trust is destroyed, how can we expect them to be happy?

Prosperity too—not so much in the sense of having an abundance of material wealth but more in the sense of flourishing mentally and emotionally—makes a significant contribution to our sense of inner peace. Here again we might think of the example of the Tibetan refugees who prospered in spite of their lack of resources.

Indeed, each of these factors plays an important part in establishing a sense of individual well-being. Yet without a basic feeling of inner peace and security, they are of no avail. Why? Because, as we saw, our possessions are themselves a source of anxiety. So are our jobs insofar as we worry about losing them. Even our friends and relatives can become a source of trouble. They may get sick and need our attention when we are busy with important business. They may even turn against us and cheat us. Similarly, our bodies, however fit and beautiful they may be at present, must eventually give in to old age. Nor are we ever invulnerable to sickness and pain. Thus there is no hope of attaining lasting happiness if we lack inner peace.

Where, then, are we to find inner peace? There is no single answer. But one thing is for sure. No external factor can create it. Nor would it be any use asking for inner peace from a doctor. The best he or she could do is offer us an antidepressant or a sleeping pill. Similarly, no machine or computer, however sophisticated and powerful, could give us this vital quality. In my view, developing inner peace, on which lasting—and therefore—meaningful happiness is dependent, is like any other task in life: we have to identify its causes and conditions and then diligently set about cultivating them. This, we find, entails a two-pronged approach. On the one hand, we need to guard against those factors which obstruct it. On the other, we need to cultivate those which are conducive to it.

So far as the conditions of inner peace are concerned, one of the most important is our basic attitude. Let me explain this by giving another personal example. Despite my habitual serenity today, I used to be somewhat hot-tempered and prone to fits of impatience and sometimes anger. Even today, there are, of course, times when I lose my composure. When this happens, the least annoyance can take on undue proportions and upset me considerably. I may, for example, wake up in the morning and feel agitated for no particular reason. In this state, I find that even what ordinarily pleases me may irritate me. Just looking at my watch can give rise to feelings of annoyance. I see it as nothing but a source of attachment and, through this, of further suffering. But then on other days I will wake up and see it as something beautiful, so intricate and delicate. Yet, of course, it is the same watch. What has changed? Are my feelings of revulsion one day and satisfaction the next purely the result of chance? Or is some neurological mechanism over which I have no control at work here? Although of course our constitution must have something to do with it, the governing factor is surely my mental attitude. Our basic attitude— how we relate to external circumstances—is thus the first consideration in any discussion on developing inner peace. In this context, the great Indian scholar-practitioner Shantideva once observed that while we have no hope of finding enough leather to cover the earth so that we never prick our feet on a thorn, actually we do not need to. As he went on to observe, enough to cover the soles of our feet will suffice. In other words, while we cannot always change our external situation to suit us, we can change our attitude.

The other major source of inner peace, and thus of genuine happiness, is, of course, the actions we undertake in our pursuit of happiness. We can classify these in terms of those which make a positive contribution toward it, those whose effect is neutral, and those which have a negative effect on it. By considering what differentiates those acts which make for lasting happiness from those which offer only a transient sense of well-being, we see that in the latter case the activities themselves have no positive value. We have a desire for something sweet, perhaps, or for some fashionable item of clothing, or to experience something new. We have no real need of it. We simply want that thing or to enjoy that experience or sensation, and we set about satisfying our craving without much thought. Now I am not suggesting there is necessarily anything wrong in this. An appetite for the concrete is part of human nature: we want to see, we want to touch, we want to possess. But, as I suggested earlier, it is essential we recognize that when we desire things for no real reason beyond the enjoyment they give us, ultimately they tend to bring us more problems. Moreover, we find that like the happiness which gratifying such perceived needs brings, they are themselves in fact transient.

We must also acknowledge that it is this very lack of concern for consequences that underlies extreme actions, like inflicting pain on others, even killing itself—either of which can certainly satisfy a person's desires for a short time—though those desires are severely negative ones. Or again, in the field of economic activity, the pursuit of profit without consideration of potentially negative consequences can undoubtedly give rise to feelings of great joy when success comes. But in the end there is suffering: the environment is polluted, our unscrupulous methods drive others out of business, the bombs we manufacture cause death and injury.

As to those activities which can lead to a sense of peace and lasting happiness, consider what happens when we do something we believe to be worthwhile. Perhaps we conceive of a plan to help our community and, eventually, after much effort, bring it to fruition. When we analyze activities of this sort, we find they involve discernment. They entail weighing different factors, including both the likely and the possible consequences for ourselves and for others. In this process of evaluation, the question of morality, of whether our intended actions are ethical, arises automatically. So while the initial impulse might be to be deceitful in order to attain some end, we reason that although we may gain temporary happiness this way, actually the long-term consequences of behaving thus are likely to bring trouble. We therefore deliberately renounce one course of action in favor of another. And it is through achieving our aim by means of effort and self-sacrifice, through considering both the short-term benefit to us and the long-term effects on others' happiness, and sacrificing the former for the latter, that we attain the happiness which is characterized by peace and by genuine satisfaction. Our differing responses to hardship confirm this. When we go on holiday, our basic motive is leisure. If, then, due to bad weather, due to clouds and rain, we are frustrated in our desire to spend time relaxing outside, our happiness is easily destroyed. On the other hand, when we seek not merely temporary satisfaction, when striving to achieve a goal, the hunger, fatigue, or discomfort we may experience hardly bothers us. In other words, altruism is an essential component of those actions which lead to genuine happiness.

There is thus an important distinction to be made between what we might call ethical and spiritual acts. An ethical act is one where we refrain from causing harm to others' experience or expectation of happiness. Spiritual acts we can describe in terms of those qualities mentioned earlier of love, compassion, patience, forgiveness, humility, tolerance, and so on which presume some level of concern for others' well-being. We find that the spiritual actions we undertake which are motivated not by narrow self-interest but out of our concern for others actually benefit ourselves. And not only that, but they make our lives meaningful. At least this is my experience. Looking back over my life, I can say with full confidence that such things as the office of Dalai Lama, the political power it confers, even the comparative wealth it puts at my disposal, contribute not even a fraction to my feelings of happiness compared with the happiness I have felt on those occasions when I have been able to benefit others.

Does this proposition stand up to analysis? Is conduct inspired by the wish to help others the most effective way to bring about genuine happiness? Consider the following. We humans are social beings. We come into the world as the result of others' actions. We survive here in dependence on others. Whether we like it or not, there is hardly a moment of our lives when we do not benefit from others' activities. For this reason, it is hardly surprising that most of our happiness arises in the context of our relationships with others. Nor is it so remarkable that our greatest joy should come when we are motivated by concern for others. But that is not all. We find that not only do altruistic actions bring about happiness, but they also lessen our experience of suffering. Here I am not suggesting that the individual whose actions are motivated by the wish to bring others' happiness necessarily meets with less misfortune than the one who does not. Sickness, old age, and mishaps of one sort or another are the same for us all. But the sufferings which undermine our internal peace—anxiety, frustration, disappointment—are definitely less. In our concern for others, we worry less about ourselves. When we worry less about ourselves, the experience of our own suffering is less intense.

What does this tell us? Firstly, because our every action has a universal dimension, a potential impact on others' happiness, ethics are necessary as a means to ensure that we do not harm others. Secondly, it tells us that genuine happiness consists in those spiritual qualities of love and compassion, patience, tolerance, forgiveness, humility, and so on. It is these which provide happiness both for ourselves and for others.

Chapter Five

THE SUPREME EMOTION

ON A RECENT TRIP TO EUROPE, I TOOK the opportunity to visit the site of the Nazi death camp at Auschwitz. Even though I had heard and read a great deal about this place, I found myself completely unprepared for the experience. My initial reaction to the sight of the ovens in which hundreds of thousands of human beings were burned was one of total revulsion. I was dumbfounded at the sheer calculation and detachment from feeling to which they bore horrifying testimony. Then, in the museum which forms part of the visitor center, I saw a collection of shoes. A lot of them were patched or small, having obviously belonged to children and poor people. This saddened me particularly. What wrong could *they* possibly have done, what harm? I stopped and prayed—moved profoundly both for the victims and for the perpetrators of this iniquity—that such a thing would never happen again. And, in the knowledge that just as we all have the capacity to act selflessly out of concern for others' well-being, so do we all have the potential to be murderers and torturers, I vowed never in any way to contribute to such a calamity.

Events such as those which occurred at Auschwitz are violent reminders of what can happen when individuals—and by extension, whole societies—lose touch with basic human feeling. But although it is necessary to have legislation and international conventions in place as safeguards against future disasters of this kind, we have all seen that atrocities continue in spite of them. Much more effective and important than such legislation is our regard for one another's feelings at a simple human level.

When I speak of basic human feeling, I am not only thinking of something fleeting and vague, however. I refer to the capacity we all have to empathize with one another, which, in Tibetan we call *shen dug ngal wa la mi sö pa*. Translated literally, this means "the inability to bear the sight of another's suffering." Given that this is what enables us to enter into, and to some extent participate, in others' pain, it is one of our most significant characteristics. It is what causes us to start at the sound of a cry for help, to recoil at the sight of harm done to another, to suffer when confronted with others' suffering. And it is what compels us to shut our eyes even when we want to ignore others' distress.

Here, imagine walking along a road, deserted save for an elderly person just ahead of you. Suddenly, that person trips and falls. What do you do? I have no doubt that the majority of readers would go over to see whether they might help. Not all, perhaps. But in admitting that not everyone would go to the assistance of another in distress, I do not mean to suggest that in those few exceptions this capacity for empathy, which I have suggested to be universal, is entirely absent. Even in the case of those who did not, surely there will at least be the same feeling, however faint, of concern, which would motivate the majority to offer their assistance? It is certainly possible to imagine people who, after enduring years of warfare, are no longer moved at the sight of others' suffering. The same could be true of those who live in places where there is an atmosphere of violence and indifference to others. It is even possible to imagine a few who would exult at the sight of another's suffering. Yet this does not prove that the capacity for empathy is not present in such people. That we all, excepting perhaps only the most disturbed, appreciate being shown kindness, suggests that however hardened we may become, the capacity for empathy remains.

This characteristic of appreciating others' concern is, I believe, a reflection of our "inability to bear the sight of another's suffering." I say this because alongside our natural ability to empathize with others, we also have a need for others' kindness, which runs like a thread throughout our whole life. It is most apparent when we are young and when we are old. But we have only to fall ill to be reminded of how important it is to be loved and cared about even during our prime years. Though it may seem a virtue to be able to do without affection, in reality a life lacking this precious ingredient must be a miserable one.

It is surely not a coincidence that the lives of most criminals turn out to have been lonely and lacking in love.

We see this appreciation of kindness reflected in our response to the human smile. For me, human beings' ability to smile is one of our most beautiful characteristics. It is something no animal can do. Not dogs, nor even whales or dolphins, each of them very intelligent beings with a clear affinity for humans, can smile as we do. Personally, I always feel a bit curious when I smile at someone and they remain serious and unresponding. On the other hand, my heart is gladdened when they reciprocate. Even in the case of someone I have nothing to do with, when that person smiles at me, I am touched. But why? The answer surely is that a genuine smile touches something fundamental in us: our natural appreciation of kindness.

Despite the body of opinion suggesting that human nature is basically aggressive and competitive, my own view is that our appreciation for affection and love is so profound that it begins even before our birth. Indeed, according to some scientist friends of mine, there is strong evidence to suggest that a mother's mental and emotional state greatly affects the well-being of her unborn child, that it benefits her baby if she maintains a warm and gentle state of mind. A happy mother bears a happy child. On the other hand, frustration and anger are harmful to the healthy development of the baby. Similarly, during the first weeks after birth, warmth and affection continue to play a supreme role in the infant's physical development. At this stage, the brain is growing very rapidly, a function which doctors believe is somehow assisted by the constant touch of the mother or surrogate. This shows that though the baby may not know or care who is who, it has a clear physical need of affection. Perhaps, too, it explains why even the most fractious, agitated, and paranoid individuals respond positively to the affection and care of others. As infants they must have been nurtured by someone. Should a baby be neglected during this critical period, clearly it could not survive.

Fortunately, this is very rarely the case. Almost without exception, the mother's first act is to offer her baby her nourishing milk—an act which to me symbolizes unconditional love. Her affection here is totally genuine and uncalculating: she expects nothing in return. As for the baby, it is drawn naturally to its mother's breast. Why? Of course we can speak of the survival instinct. But in addition I think it reasonable to conjecture a degree of affection on the part of the infant toward its mother. If it felt aversion, surely it would not suckle? And if the mother felt aversion, it is doubtful her milk would flow freely. What we see instead is a relationship based on love and mutual tenderness, which is totally spontaneous. It is not learned from others, no religion requires it, no laws impose it, no schools have taught it. It arises quite naturally.

This instinctual care of mother for child— shared it seems with many animals—is crucial because it suggests that alongside the baby's fundamental need of love in order to survive, there exists an innate capacity on the part of the mother to give love. So powerful is it that we might almost suppose a biological component is at work. Of course it could be argued that this reciprocal love is nothing more than a survival mechanism. That could well be so. But that is not to deny its existence. Nor indeed does it undermine my conviction that this need and capacity for love suggest that we are, in fact, loving by nature.

If this seems improbable, consider our differing response to kindness and to violence. Most of us find violence intimidating. Conversely, when we are shown kindness, we respond with greater trust. Similarly, consider the relationship between peace—which as we have seen is the fruit of love—and good health. According to my understanding, our constitution is more suited to peace and tranquility than to violence and aggression. We all know that stress and anxiety can lead to high blood pressure and other negative symptoms. In the Tibetan medical system, mental and emotional disturbances are considered to be a cause of many constitutional diseases, including cancer. Moreover, peace, tranquility, and others' care are essential to recovery from illness. We can also identify a basic longing for peace. Why? Because peace suggests life and growth whereas violence suggests only misery and death. This is why the idea of a Pure Land, or of Heaven, attracts us. If such a place were described in terms of unending warfare and strife, we would much rather remain in this world.

Notice, too, how we respond to the phenomenon of life itself. When spring follows winter, the days become longer, there is more sunshine, the grass grows afresh: automatically our spirits lift. On the other hand, at the approach of winter, the leaves begin to fall one by one, and much of the vegetation around us becomes as though dead. Small wonder if we tend to feel a bit downcast at that time of year. The indication here is surely that our nature prefers life over death, growth over decay, construction over destruction.

Consider also the behavior of children. In them we see what is natural to the human character before it has been overlaid with learned ideas. We find that very young babies do not really differentiate between one person and another. They attach much more importance to the smile of the person in front of them than to anything else. Even when they start to grow up, they are not very interested in differences of race, nationality, religion, or family background. When they meet with other children, they do not stop to discuss these things. They immediately begin the much more important business of play. Nor is this just sentimentalism. I see the reality whenever I visit one of the children's villages in Europe, where numbers of Tibetan refugee children have been educated since the early 1960s. These villages were founded to care for orphaned children from countries at war with one another. To no one's great surprise, it was found that despite their different backgrounds, when these children are put together, they live in complete harmony with one another.

Now it could be objected that while we may all share a capacity for loving-kindness, human nature is such that inevitably we tend to reserve it for those closest to us. We are biased toward our families and friends. Our feelings of concern for those outside the circle will depend very much on individual circumstances: those who feel threatened are not likely to have very much goodwill for those who threaten them. All this is true enough. Nor do I deny that whatever our capacity to feel concern for our fellow human beings, when our very survival is threatened, it may but rarely prevail over the instinct for self-preservation. Still, this does not mean that the capacity is no longer there, that the potential does not remain. Even soldiers after a battle will often help their enemies retrieve their dead and wounded.

In all of what I have said about our basic nature, I do not mean to suggest that I believe it has no negative aspects. Where there is consciousness, hatred, ignorance, and violence do indeed arise naturally. This is why, although our nature is basically disposed toward kindness and compassion, we are all capable of cruelty and hatred. It is why we have to struggle

72

to better our conduct. It also explains how individuals raised in a strictly non-violent environment have turned into the most horrible butchers. In connection with this, I recall my visit some years ago to the Washington Memorial, which pays tribute to the martyrs and heroes of the Jewish Holocaust at the hands of the Nazis. What struck me most forcefully about the monument was its simultaneous cataloging of different forms of human behavior. On one side it lists the victims of acts of unspeakable atrocity. On the other, it remembers the heroic acts of kindness on the part of Christian families and others who willingly took terrible risks in order to harbor their Jewish brothers and sisters. I felt that this was entirely appropriate, and very necessary: to show the two sides of human potential.

But the existence of this negative potential does not give us grounds to suppose that human nature is inherently violent, or even necessarily disposed toward violence. Perhaps one of the reasons for the popularity of the belief that human nature is aggressive lies in our continual exposure to bad news through the media. Yet the very cause of this is surely that good news is not news.

To say that basic human nature is not only non-violent but actually disposed toward love and compassion, kindness, gentleness, affection, creation, and so on does, of course, imply a general principle which must, by definition, be applicable to each individual human being. What, then, are we to say about those individuals whose lives seem to be given over wholly to violence and aggression? During the past century alone there are several obvious examples to consider. What of Hitler and his plan to exterminate the entire Jewish race? What of Stalin and his pogroms? What of Chairman Mao, the man I once knew and admired, and the barbarous insanity of the Cultural Revolution? What of Pol Pot, architect of the Killing Fields? And what about those who torture and kill for pleasure?

Here I must admit that I can think of no single explanation to account for the monstrous acts of these people. However, we must recognize two things. Firstly, such people do not come from nowhere but from within a particular society at a particular time and in a particular place. Their actions need to be considered in relation to these circumstances. Secondly, we need to recognize the role of the imaginative faculty in their actions. Their schemes were and are carried out in accordance with a vision, albeit a perverted one. Notwithstanding the fact that nothing could justify the suffering they instigated, whatever their explanation might be and whatever positive intentions they could point to, Hitler, Stalin, Mao, and Pol Pot each had goals toward which they were working. If we examine those actions which are uniquely human, which animals cannot perform, we find that this imaginative faculty plays a vital role. The faculty itself is a unique asset. But the use to which it is put determines whether the actions it conceives are positive or negative, ethical or unethical. The individual's motivation (*kun long*) is thus the governing factor. And whereas a vision properly motivated—which recognizes others' desire for and equal right to happiness and to be free of suffering—can lead to wonders, when divorced from basic human feeling the potential for destruction cannot be overestimated.

As for those who kill for pleasure or, worse, for no reason at all, we can only conjecture a deep submergence of the basic impulse toward care and affection for others. Still this need not mean that it is entirely extinguished. As I pointed out earlier, except perhaps in the most extreme cases, it is possible to imagine even these people appreciating being shown affection. The disposition remains.

Actually, the reader does not need to accept my proposition that human nature is basically disposed toward love and compassion to see that the capacity for empathy which underlies it is of crucial importance when it comes to ethics. We saw earlier how an ethical act is a non-harming act. But how are we to determine whether an act is genuinely non-harming? We find that in practice, if we are not able to connect with others to some extent, if we cannot at least imagine the potential impact of our actions on others, then we have no means to discriminate between right and wrong, between what is appropriate and what is not, between harming and non-harming. It follows, therefore, that if we could enhance this capacity—that is to say, our sensitivity toward others' suffering—the more we did so, the less we could tolerate seeing others' pain and the more we would be concerned to ensure that no action of ours caused harm to others.

The fact that we can indeed enhance our capacity for empathy becomes obvious when we consider its nature. We experience it mainly as a feeling. And, as we all know, to a greater or lesser extent we can not only restrain our feelings through reasoning, but we can enhance them in the same way. Our desire for objects—perhaps a new car—is enhanced by our turning it over and over in our imagination. Similarly, when, as it were, we direct our mental faculties onto our feelings of empathy, we find that not only can we enhance them, but we can transform them into love and compassion itself.

As such, our innate capacity for empathy is the source of that most precious of all human qualities, which in Tibetan we call *nying je*. Now while generally translated simply as "compassion," the term *nying je* has a wealth of meaning that is difficult to convey succinctly, though the ideas it contains are universally understood. It connotes love, affection, kindness, gentleness, generosity of spirit, and warm-heartedness. It is also used as a term of both sympathy and of endearment. On the other hand, it does not imply "pity" as the word compassion may. There is no sense of condescension. On the contrary, *nying je* denotes a feeling of connection with others, reflecting its origins in empathy. Thus while we might say, "I love my house" or "I have strong feelings of affection for this place," we cannot say, "I have compassion" for these things. Having no feelings themselves, we cannot empathize with objects. We cannot, therefore, speak of having compassion for them.

Although it is clear from this description that *nying je*, or love and compassion, is understood as an emotion, it belongs to that category of emotions which have a more developed cognitive component. Some emotions, such as the revulsion we tend to feel at the sight of blood, are basically instinctual. Others, such as fear of poverty, have this more developed cognitive component. We can thus understand *nying je* in terms of a combination of empathy and reason. We can think of empathy as the characteristic of a very honest person; reason as that of someone who is very practical. When the two are put together, the combination is highly effective. As such, *nying je* is quite different from those random feelings, like anger and lust, which, far from bringing us happiness, only trouble us and destroy our peace of mind.

To me, this suggests that by means of sustained reflection on, and familiarization with, compassion, through rehearsal and practice we can develop our innate ability to connect with others, a fact which is of supreme importance given the approach to ethics I have described. The more we develop compassion, the more genuinely ethical our conduct will be.

As we have seen, when we act out of concern for others, our behavior toward them is automatically positive. This is because we have no room for suspicion when our hearts are filled with love. It is as if an inner door is opened, allowing us to reach out. Having concern for others breaks down the very barriers which inhibit healthy interaction with others. And not only that. When our intentions toward others are good, we find that any feelings of shyness or insecurity we may have are greatly reduced. To the extent that we are able to open this inner door, we experience a sense of liberation from our habitual preoccupation with self. Paradoxically, we find this gives rise to strong feelings of confidence. Thus, if I may give an example from my own experience, I find that whenever I meet new people and have this positive disposition, there is no barrier between us. No matter who or what they are, whether they have blond hair or black hair, or hair dyed green, I feel that I am simply encountering a fellow human being with the same desire to be happy and to avoid suffering as myself. And I find I can speak to them as if they were old friends, even at our first meeting. By keeping in mind that ultimately we are all brothers and sisters, that there is no substantial difference between us, that just as I do, all others share my desire to be happy and to avoid suffering, I can express my feelings as readily as to someone I have known intimately for years. And not just with a few nice words or gestures but really heart to heart, no matter what the language barrier.

We also find that when we act out of concern for others, the peace this creates in our own hearts brings peace to everyone we associate with. We bring peace to the family, peace to our friends, to the workplace, to the community, and so to the world. Why, then, would anyone not wish to develop this quality? Could anything be more sublime than that which brings peace and happiness to all? For my own part, the mere ability we human beings have to sing the praises of love and compassion is a most precious gift.

Conversely, not even the most skeptical reader could suppose that peace ever comes about as the result of aggressive and inconsiderate, that is to say, unethical behavior. Of course it cannot. I well remember how I learned this particular lesson when I was a small boy in Tibet. One of my attendants, Kenrab Tenzin, had made a pet of a small parrot, which he used to feed with nuts. Although he was a rather stern man with bulging eyes and a somewhat forbidding aspect, merely at the sound of his footsteps, or of his coughing, this parrot would show signs of excitement. As the bird nibbled from his fingers, Kenrab Tenzin would stroke its head, which appeared to put it into a state of ecstasy. I was very envious of this relationship and desired the bird to show me the same friendliness. But when I tried on a few occasions to feed it myself, I failed to get a good response. So I tried poking at it with a stick in the hope of provoking a better reaction. Needless to say, the result was totally negative. Far from forcing it to behave better toward me, the bird took fright. What little prospect of establishing friendly relations there may have been was totally destroyed. I learned thereby that friendships come about not as the result of bullying but as a result of compassion.

The world's major religious traditions each give the development of compassion a key role. Because it is both the source and the result of patience, tolerance, forgiveness, and all good qualities, its importance is considered to extend from the beginning to the end of spiritual practice. But even without a religious perspective, love and compassion are clearly of fundamental importance to us all. Given our basic premise that ethical conduct consists in not harming others, it follows that we need to take others' feelings into consideration, the basis for which is our innate capacity for empathy. And as we transform this capacity into love and compassion, through guarding against those factors which obstruct compassion and cultivating those conducive to it, so our practice of ethics improves. This, we find, leads to happiness both for ourselves and others.

II

Ethics and the Individual

Chapter Six

THE ETHIC OF RESTRAINT

I HAVE SUGGESTED THAT DEVELOPING THE compassion on which happiness depends demands a two-pronged approach. On the one hand, we need to restrain those factors which inhibit compassion. On the other, we need to cultivate those which are conducive to it. As we have seen, what is conducive to compassion is love, patience, tolerance, forgiveness, humility, and so on. What inhibits compassion is that lack of inner restraint which we have identified as the source of all unethical conduct. We find that by transforming our habits and dispositions, we can begin to perfect our overall state of heart and mind (*kun long*)—that from which all our actions spring.

The first thing, then—because the spiritual qualities conducive to compassion entail positive ethical conduct—is to cultivate a habit of inner discipline. Now I cannot deny that this is a major undertaking, but at least we are familiar with the principle. For example, knowing its destructive potential, we restrain both ourselves and our children from indulging in drug abuse. However, it is important to recognize that restraining our response to negative thoughts and emotions is not a matter of just suppressing them: insight into their destructive nature is crucial. Merely being told that envy, potentially a very powerful and destructive emotion, is negative cannot provide a strong defense against it. If we order our lives externally but ignore the inner dimension, inevitably we will find that doubt, anxiety, and other afflictions develop, and happiness eludes us. This is because, unlike physical discipline, true inner—or spiritual—discipline cannot be achieved by force but only through voluntary and deliberate effort based on understanding. In other words, conducting ourselves ethically consists in more than merely obeying laws and precepts.

The undisciplined mind is like an elephant. If left to blunder around out of control, it will wreak havoc. But the harm and suffering we encounter as a result of failing to restrain the negative impulses of mind far exceed the damage a rampaging elephant can cause. Not only are these impulses capable of bringing about the destruction of things, they can also be the cause of lasting pain to others and to ourselves. By this I do not mean to suggest that the mind (*lo*) is inherently destructive. Under the influence of a strongly negative thought or emotion, the mind may seem to be characterized by a single quality. But if, for instance, hatefulness were an unchangeable characteristic of consciousness, then consciousness must always be hateful. Clearly this is not the case. There is an important distinction to be made between consciousness as such and the thoughts and emotions it experiences.

Similarly, while at the time a powerful experience may overwhelm us, when we consider it later, we are unmoved. When very young, I used to become highly excited, as the old year drew to a close, at the thought of *monlam chenmo*. This was the Great Prayer Festival which marked the start of the Tibetan New Year. In my capacity as Dalai Lama, I had an important role in this, which meant moving from the Potala to a set of rooms in the Jokhang temple, one of Tibet's holiest shrines. As the day drew closer, I would spend more and more time daydreaming at the prospect, half-terrified and half-elated, and less and less time studying. My feelings of terror were caused by the thought of the long recital I had to give from memory during the main ceremony, my excitement by the thought of passing among the huge crowd of pilgrims and traders thronging the market place in front of the temple complex. Even though both the overexcitement and the aversion I felt were real enough then, today, of course, I can laugh at these memories. I am now quite used to crowds.And, after so many years of practice, the recitation no longer troubles me.

We can conceive the nature of mind in terms of the water in a lake. When the water is stirred up by a storm, the mud from the lake's bottom clouds it, making it appear opaque. But the nature of the water is not dirty. When the storm passes, the mud settles and the water is left clear once again. So although generally we may suppose mind, or consciousness, to be an inherent and unchangeable entity, when we consider it more deeply, we see that it consists in a whole spectrum of events and experiences. These include our sensory perception, which engages with objects directly, as well as our thoughts and feelings, which are mediated by language and concepts. It is also dynamic: through deliberate engagement we can effect changes in our mental and emotional states. We know, for example, how comfort and reassurance can help dispel fear. Similarly, those forms of counseling which lead to greater awareness, and affection, can help alleviate depression.

This observation, that emotion and consciousness are not the same thing, tells us that we do not have to be controlled by our thoughts and emotions. Prior to our every action, there must be a mental and emotional event to which we are more or less free to respond, albeit that until we have learned to discipline our mind, we will have difficulty in exercising this freedom. Again, how we respond to these events and experiences is moreover that which determines the moral content of our acts, generally speaking. In simple terms, this means that if we do so positively, keeping others' interests before us, our acts will be positive. If we respond negatively, neglecting others, our acts will be negative and unethical.

According to this understanding, we might think of mind, or consciousness, in terms of a president or monarch who is very honest, very pure. In this view, our thoughts and emotions are like cabinet ministers. Some of them give good advice, some bad. Some have the well-being of others as their principal concern, others only their own narrow interests. The responsibility of the main consciousness—the leader—is to determine which of these subordinates gives good advice and which bad, which of them are reliable and which are not, and to act on the advice of the one sort and not the other.

Mental and emotional events which, in this sense, give bad advice can themselves be described as a form of suffering. Indeed, we find that when they are allowed to develop to any significant degree, the mind becomes swamped with emotion, and we experience a kind of inner turbulence. This also has a physical dimension. In a moment of anger, for example, we experience a powerful disturbance of our habitual equilibrium, which can often be sensed by others. We are all familiar with the way in which the whole atmosphere is spoiled when just one member of the household is in a bad mood. When we become enraged, both people and animals tend to avoid us. Sometimes this turbulence is so strong that we find great difficulty containing it. This can cause us to lash out at others. In doing so, we externalize our inner turbulence.

This is not to say that all thoughts and emotions which cause us discomfort are necessarily negative. The primary attribute that distinguishes ordinary emotions from those which undermine peace is its negative cognitive component. A moment of sorrow does not become disabling grief unless we hold on to it and add negative thoughts and imaginings. In the case both of the overexcitement I felt about those crowds of pilgrims and traders and the fear I had of the long recitation, there was an added cognitive component on top of the basic feeling. Through my somewhat obsessive daydreaming, my imagination superimposed something beyond the reality of the situation. And it was the stories I told myself about the forthcoming event that undermined my basic serenity.

Nor is all fear like the childish one I have just described. There are occasions when we experience a more rational kind of fear. Far from being negative, this may actually be helpful. It can heighten our awareness and give us the energy we need to protect ourselves. On the first night of my escape from Lhasa in 1959, when I left home dressed as a soldier, I certainly felt this kind of fear. But because I had neither the time nor the inclination to think about it, it did not unsettle me very much. Its main effect was to make me very alert. One could say that this was an instance of fear which was both justified and useful.

The fear we feel in relation to a situation which is quite delicate or critical may also be justified. Here I am thinking of what we feel when we have to make a decision we know will have a significant impact on others' lives. Such fear may disconcert us somewhat. But the most dangerous and negative is that fear which is completely unreasonable and which can totally overwhelm and paralyze us.

In Tibetan, we call such negative and emotional events *nyong mong*, literally, "that which afflicts from within" or, as the term is usually translated, "afflictive emotion." On this view, generally speaking, all those thoughts, emotions, and mental events which reflect a negative or uncompassionate state of mind (*kun long*) inevitably undermine our experience of inner peace. All negative thoughts and emotions—such as hatred, anger, pride, lust, greed, envy, and so on—are considered to be afflictions in this sense. We find that these afflictive emotions are so strong that if we do nothing to counter them, though there is no one who does not value their life, they can lead us to the point of madness and even suicide itself. But because such extremes are unusual, we tend to see negative emotions as an integral part of our mind about which we can do very little. And, in failing to recognize their destructive potential, we do not see the need to challenge them. Indeed, far from doing so, we have a tendency to nurture and reinforce them. This provides them the ground in which to grow. Yet, as we shall see, their nature is wholly destructive. They are the very source of unethical conduct. They are also the basis of anxiety, depression, confusion, and stress, which are such a feature of our lives today.

Negative thoughts and emotions are what obstruct our most basic aspiration—to be happy and to avoid suffering. When we act under their influence, we become oblivious to the impact our actions have on others: they are thus the cause of our destructive behavior both toward others and to ourselves. Murder, scandal, and deceit all have their origin in afflictive emotion. This is why I say that the undisciplined mind—that is, the mind under the influence of anger, hatred, greed, pride, selfishness, and so on—is the source of all our troubles which do not fall into the category of unavoidable suffering (sickness, old age, death, and so on). Our failure to check our response to the afflictive emotions opens the door to suffering for both self and others.

To say that when we cause others to suffer we ourselves suffer does not, of course, mean we can logically infer that in every instance when, for example, I hit someone, I will be hit myself. The proposition I am making is much more general than this. Rather, I mean to suggest that the impact of our actions—both positive and negative—registers deep within us. If it is correct that, on some level, we all have the capacity for empathy, it follows that for one individual to harm another, this potential must be overwhelmed, or submerged in some way. Take the case of a person who cruelly tortures another. Their mind (*lo*) must be strongly gripped at the gross, or conscious level, by some kind of harmful thinking or ideology which causes them to believe their victim is deserving of such treatment. Such a belief—which to some degree must have been deliberately chosen—is what enables the cruel person to suppress their feelings. Nevertheless, deep down, there is bound to be some kind of effect. In the long run, there is a high degree of probability that discomfort will be felt by the torturer. Consider in this context the example we looked at earlier—of merciless dictators like Hitler and Stalin. It seems that as they neared the end of their lives, they became lonely, anxious, full of dread, and suspicion, like crows afraid of their own shadows.

Of course, the number of people who go to such extremes is very small. The impact of minor negative actions is also much more subtle than major ones. So, as a less extreme example of the way in which negative actions cause suffering both to ourselves as well as others, consider a child going out to play who gets into a fight with another child. Immediately after, the victorious child may experience a sense of satisfaction. But on returning home, that emotion will subside and a more subtle state of mind will manifest. At that point, a sense of unease sets in. We could almost describe this sort of feeling as a sense of alienation from self: the individual doesn't feel quite "right." In the contrary case of a child who goes out to play and shares an enjoyable afternoon with a friend, afterwards not only will there be an immediate sense of satisfaction, but when the mind has settled down and the excitement worn off, there will be a sense of calm and comfort.

Another example of the way in which negative actions harm the one who indulges them can be seen in the context of an individual's reputation. Generally, it seems, we humans— even, for that matter, animals—abhor meanness, aggressiveness, deceit, and so on. To me this suggests that if we engage in activities which harm others, despite the temporary satisfaction we might gain thereby, people will at some point begin to look at us askance. They will become apprehensive of us, nervous and suspicious on account of our bad reputation. In time, we will start to lose friends. In this way, because a good reputation is a source of happiness, we bring suffering on ourselves if we spoil it.

Indeed, though there may be a few exceptions, we find that if a person lives a very selfish life, without concern for others' welfare, they tend to become quite lonely and miserable. Though they may be surrounded by people who are friends of their wealth or status, when the selfish or aggressive individual faces tragedy, not only do these so-called friends vanish, they may even secretly rejoice. And if, moreover, he or she is actively malicious, it is likely that when they die they are not much missed. People may actually be glad—as many of the inmates of the Nazi death camps must have been at the subsequent execution of their captors. Conversely, we find that when people are actively concerned for others, they are much respected, even venerated. When such people die, many mourn and regret their passing. Consider the case of Mahatma Gandhi. Despite a Western education and despite the opportunities this gave him to lead a comfortable life, he chose out of consideration for others to live in India almost as a beggar in order to devote himself to his life's work. Yet though his name is now just a memory, millions still draw comfort and inspiration from his noble deeds.

As far as the actual cause of afflictive emotion is concerned, we can point to a number of different factors. These include the habit we all have of thinking of ourselves before others. We can also cite our tendency to project characteristics onto things and events above and beyond what actually is there—as in the example of mistaking the coiled rope for a snake. But beyond these, because our negative thoughts and emotions do not exist independently of other phenomena, the very objects and events we come into contact with play a role in shaping our responses. There is thus nothing which does not have the potential to trigger them. Anything can be a source of afflictive emotion— not just our adversaries but our friends and our most valued possessions, too, even our own selves.

This suggests that the first step in the process of actually countering our negative thoughts and emotions is to avoid those situations and activities which would normally give rise to them. If, for example, we find we become angry whenever we meet with a particular person, it may be best to keep away from them until we develop our internal resources more. The second step is to avoid the actual conditions which lead to these strong thoughts and emotions. This, however, presupposes that we have learned to recognize afflictive emotions as they arise in us. This is not always easy. While hatred is a very strong emotion when fully developed, in its beginning stages the aversion we feel toward a particular object or event may be quite subtle. And even at their most advanced stages of development, afflictive emotions do not always manifest dramatically. The assassin may be relatively calm in the moment that he pulls the trigger.

To this end, we need to pay close attention and be aware of our body and its actions, of our speech and what we say, and of our hearts and minds and what we think and feel. We must be on the lookout for the slightest negativity and keep asking ourselves such questions as, "Am I happier when my thoughts and emotions are negative and destructive or when they are wholesome?" "What is the nature of consciousness? Does it exist in and of itself, or does it exist in dependence on other factors?" We need to think, think, think. We should be like a scientist who collects data, analyzes it, and draws the appropriate conclusion. Gaining insight into our own negativity is a lifelong task, and one which is capable of almost infinite refinement. But unless we undertake it, we will be unable to see where to make the necessary changes in our lives.

Were we to expend even a fraction of the time and effort we consume in trivial activities—pointless gossip and the like—on gaining insight into the actual nature of afflictive emotion, I believe it would have a huge impact on our quality of life. Both individuals and society would benefit. One of the first things we would discover is how destructive afflictive emotions are. And the more we develop an appreciation of their destructive nature, the more disinclined we would become to follow them. This alone would have a significant impact on our lives.

Consider that not only do negative thoughts and emotions destroy our experience of peace, they also undermine our health. In the Tibetan medical system, anger is a primary source of many illnesses, including those associated with high blood pressure, sleeplessness, and degenerative disorders—a view which seems increasingly accepted in allopathic medicine.

Another childhood memory illustrates the way in which afflictive emotions harm us. When I was a teenager, one of my favorite pastimes was tinkering with the old cars that my predecessor, the Thirteenth Dalai Lama, had acquired not long before he died in 1933. There were four of them, two baby Austins of British manufacture, a Dodge, and a beat-up jeep, both of American origin. Together they comprised almost the only powered vehicles in Tibet. For the young Dalai Lama, these dusty relics held an irresistible attraction, and I longed to have them running again.

My secret dream was actually to learn to drive. But it was only after a lot of pestering of various government officials that finally I found someone who knew anything about cars. This was Lhakpa Tsering, who came from Kalimpong, a town just over the Indian border. One day, I recall, he was working on the engine of one of the cars when, dropping his spanner, he shouted an oath and stood up abruptly. Unfortunately, he had forgotten the hood open above him and he hit his head with a terrible crack. But then to my great surprise, instead of extracting himself carefully, he become further enraged, and, straightening up again, hit his head even harder a second time. For a moment, I stood astonished at these antics. Then I found I could not stop laughing.

Lhakpa Tsering's outburst resulted in nothing more than two generous bruises. That was merely unfortunate for him. But from this we see how the afflictive emotions destroy one of our most precious qualities, namely, our capacity for discriminative awareness. Robbed of what enables us to judge between right and wrong, to evaluate what is likely to be of lasting benefit and what of merely temporary benefit to self and others, and to discern the likely outcome of our actions, we are no better off than animals. Small wonder that under their influence we do what ordinarily we would never consider doing.

This obliteration of our critical faculties points to another negative characteristic of this type of mental and emotional event. Afflictive emotions deceive us. They seem to offer satisfaction. But they do not provide it. In fact, although such emotion comes to us in the guise of a protector giving us, as it were, boldness and strength, we find that this energy is essentially blind. Decisions taken under its influence are often a source of regret. More often than not, such anger is actually an indication of weakness rather than of strength. Most people have experienced an argument deteriorating to the point where one person becomes verbally abusive, a clear sign of the fragility of their position. Moreover, we do not need anger to develop courage and confidence. As we shall see, it can be done through other means.

The afflictive emotions also have an irrational dimension. They encourage us to suppose that appearances are invariably commensurate with reality. When we become angry or feel hatred, we tend to relate to others as if their characteristics were immutable. A person can appear to be objectionable from the crown of their head to the soles of their feet. We forget that they, like us, are merely suffering human beings with the same wish to be happy and to avoid suffering as we ourselves. Yet common sense alone tells us that when the force of our anger diminishes, they are sure to seem a little better at least. The same is true in reverse when individuals become infatuated. The other appears to be wholly desirable—until such time as the grip of afflictive emotion subsides and they come to seem a little less than perfect. Indeed, when our passions become so strongly aroused, there is considerable danger of going to the opposite extreme. The individual once idolized now seems despicable and hateful, though of course it is the same person throughout.

The afflictive emotions are also useless. The more we give in to them, the less room we have for our good qualities—for kindness and compassion—and the less able we are to solve our problems. Indeed, there is no occasion when these disturbing thoughts and emotions are helpful either to ourselves or to others. The more angry we are, the more people shun us. The more suspicious we are, the more cut off from people we become and thus the more lonely. The more lustful we are, the less we are able to develop proper relationships with others and, again, the more lonely we become. Consider the individual whose activities are directed principally by afflictive emotion or, to put it another way, by gross attachments and aversions: by greed, arrogant ambition, and so forth. Such a person may become very powerful and very famous. Their name may even go down in history. But after they die, their power is gone and their fame is no more than an empty word. So what have they really achieved?

Nowhere is the uselessness of afflictive emotion more obvious than in the case of anger. When we become angry, we stop being compassionate, loving, generous, forgiving, tolerant, and patient altogether. We thus deprive ourselves of the very things that happiness consists in. And not only does anger immediately destroy our critical faculties, it tends toward rage, spite, hatred, and malice—each of which is always negative because it is a direct cause of harm for others. Anger causes suffering. At the very least, it causes the pain of embarrassment. For example, I have always enjoyed repairing watches. But I can recall a number of occasions as a boy when, completely losing my patience with those tiny, intricate parts, I picked up the mechanism and smashed it down on the table. Of course, later I felt very sorry and ashamed of my behavior— especially when, as on one occasion, I had to return the watch to its owner in a condition worse than it was before!

This story, trivial in itself, also makes the point that though we may have an abundance of material wealth—good food, fine furnishings, a nice television set—when we become angry, we lose all inner peace. We no longer enjoy even our breakfast. And when it becomes habitual, we may be ever so learned, rich, or powerful, but others will simply avoid us. They will say, "Oh, yes, he is very clever, but he has such bad moods, you know," and people will keep away. Or they will say, "Yes she is extraordinarily talented, but she gets upset so easily. You had better watch out." Just as when a dog is always growling and showing its teeth, we are cautious of those whose hearts are disturbed by anger. We would rather forgo their company than risk an outburst.

I do not deny that, as in the case of fear, there is a kind of "raw" anger that we experience more as a rush of energy than as a cognitively enhanced emotion. Conceivably, this form of anger could have positive consequences. It is not impossible to imagine anger at the sight of injustice causing someone to act altruistically. The anger that causes us to go to the assistance of someone who is being attacked in the street could be characterized as positive. But if this goes beyond meeting the injustice, if it becomes personal and turns into vengefulness or maliciousness, then danger arises. When we do something negative, we are capable of recognizing the difference between ourselves and the negative act. But we often fail to separate action and agent when it comes to others. This shows us how unreliable is even apparently justified anger.

Should it still seem too much to say that anger is an entirely useless emotion, we can ask ourselves if anyone ever says anger can bring happiness? No one does. What doctor prescribes anger as treatment for any disease? There isn't one. Anger can only hurt us. It has nothing to recommend it. Let the reader ask himself or herself: when we become angry, do we feel happy? Does our mind become calmer and our body relax? Or rather is it not that we feel tense in body and unsettled of mind?

If we are to retain our peace of mind and thereby our happiness, it follows that alongside a more rational and disinterested approach to our negative thoughts and emotions, we must cultivate a strong habit of restraint in response to them. Negative thoughts and emotions are what cause us to act unethically. Furthermore, because afflictive emotion is also the source of our own internal suffering— in that it is the basis of frustration, confusion, insecurity, anxiety, and the very loss of self-respect which undermines our sense of confidence—failure to do so means that we will remain in a state of perpetual mental and emotional discomfort. Inner peace will be impossible. In place of happiness there will be insecurity. Anxiety and depression will never be far away.

Some people feel that although it may be right to curb those feelings of intense hatred which can cause us to be violent and even to kill, we are in danger of losing our independence when we restrain our emotions and discipline the mind. Actually, the opposite is true. Like their counterparts of love and compassion, anger and the afflictive emotions can never be used up. They have, rather, a propensity to increase, like a river flooding in summer when the snow melts, so that far from being free, our minds are enslaved and rendered helpless by them. When we indulge our negative thoughts and feelings, inevitably we become accustomed to them. As a result, gradually we become more prone to them and more controlled by them. And we become habituated to exploding in the face of displeasing circumstances.

Inner peace, which is the principal characteristic of happiness, and anger cannot coexist without undermining one another. Indeed, negative thoughts and emotions undermine the very causes of peace and happiness. In fact, when we think properly, it is totally illogical to seek happiness if we do nothing to restrain angry, spiteful, and malicious thoughts and emotions. Consider that when we become angry, we often use harsh words. Harsh words can destroy friendship. Since happiness arises in the context of our relationships with others, if we destroy friendships, we undermine one of the very conditions of happiness itself.

To say that we need to curb anger and our negative thoughts and emotions does not mean that we should deny our feelings. There is an important distinction to be made between denial and restraint. The latter constitutes a deliberate and voluntarily adopted discipline based on an appreciation of the benefits of doing so. This is very different from the case of someone who suppresses emotions such as anger out of a feeling that they need to present a façade of self-control, or out of fear of what others may think. Such behavior is like closing a wound which is still infected. We are not talking about rule-following. Where denial and suppression occur, there comes the danger that in so doing the individual stores up anger and resentment. The trouble here is that at some future point they may find they cannot contain these feelings any longer.

In other words, there are, of course, thoughts and emotions which it is appropriate, even important, to express openly—including negative ones—albeit there are more or less appropriate ways to do so. It is far better to confront a person or situation than to hide our anger away, brood on it, and nurture resentment in our hearts. Yet if we indiscriminately express negative thoughts and emotions simply on the grounds that they must be articulated, there is a strong possibility, for all the reasons I have given, that we will lose control and overreact. Thus the important thing is to be discriminating, both in terms of the feelings we express and in how we express them.

As I understand it, genuine happiness is characterized by inner peace and arises in the context of our relationships with others. It therefore depends on ethical conduct. This in turn consists in acts which take others' well-being into account. What obstructs us from engaging in such compassionate conduct is afflictive emotion. If, then, we wish to be happy, we need to curb our response to negative thoughts and emotions. This is what I mean when I say that we must tame the wild elephant that is the undisciplined mind. When I fail to restrain my response to afflictive emotion, my actions become unethical and obstruct the causes of my happiness. We are not talking about attaining Buddhahood here, we are not talking about achieving union with God. We are merely recognizing that my interests and future happiness are closely connected to others' and learning to act accordingly.

Chapter Seven

THE ETHIC OF VIRTUE

I HAVE SUGGESTED THAT IF WE ARE TO be genuinely happy, inner restraint is indispensable. We cannot stop at restraint, however. Though it may prevent us from performing any grossly negative misdeeds, mere restraint is insufficient if we are to attain that happiness which is characterized by inner peace. In order to transform ourselves—our habits and dispositions—so that our actions are compassionate, it is necessary to develop what we might call an *ethic of virtue*. As well as refraining from negative thoughts and emotions, we need to cultivate and reinforce our positive qualities. What are these positive qualities? Our basic human, or spiritual, qualities.

After compassion (*nying je*) itself, the chief of these is what in Tibetan we call *sö pa*. Once again, we have a term which appears to have no ready equivalent in other languages, though the ideas it conveys are universal.

Often, *sö pa* is translated simply as "patience," though its literal meaning is "able to bear" or "able to withstand." But the word also carries a notion of resolution. It thus denotes a deliberate response (as opposed to an unreasoned reaction) to the strong negative thoughts and emotions that tend to arise when we encounter harm. As such, *sö pa* is what provides us with the strength to resist suffering and protects us from losing compassion even for those who would harm us.

In this context, I am reminded of the example of Lopon-la, a monk from Namgyal monastery. Following my escape from Tibet, Lopon-la was one of many thousands of monks and officials imprisoned by the occupying forces. When he was finally released, he was allowed to come to India, where he rejoined his old monastery now refounded in exile. More than twenty years after last seeing him, I found Lopon-la much as I remembered him. He looked older, of course, but physically he was unscathed, and mentally his ordeal had not affected him adversely at all. His gentleness and serenity remained. From our conversation, I learned that he had, nevertheless, endured grievous treatment during those long years of imprisonment. In common with all others, he had been subjected to "re-education," during which he had been forced to denounce his religion, and, on many occasions, he was tortured as well. When I asked him whether he had ever been afraid, he admitted that there was one thing that had scared him:

the possibility that he might lose compassion and concern for his jailers.

I was very moved by this, and also very inspired. Hearing Lopon-la's story confirmed what I had always believed. It is not just a person's physical constitution, nor their intelligence, nor their education, nor even their social conditioning which enables them to withstand hardship. Much more significant is their spiritual state. And while some may be able to survive through sheer willpower, the ones who suffer the least are those who attain a high level of *sö pa*.

Forbearance and also fortitude (courage in the face of adversity) are two words which come quite close to describing *sö pa* at its first level. But when a person develops it more, there comes composure in adversity, a sense of being unperturbed, reflecting a voluntary acceptance of hardship in pursuit of a higher, spiritual, aim. This involves accepting the reality of a given situation through recognizing that underlying its particularity, there is a vastly complex web of interrelated causes and conditions.

Sö pa is thus the means by which we practice true non-violence. It is what enables us not only to refrain from physical reactions when we are provoked, but it enables us to let go of our negative thoughts and emotions too. We cannot speak of *sö pa* when we give in to someone yet we do so grudgingly or resentfully. If, for example, a superior in the workplace upsets us yet we are obliged to defer to them despite our feelings, that is not *sö pa*. The essence of *sö pa* is resolute forbearance in the face of adversity. In other words, the one who practices patient forbearance is determined not to give in to negative impulses (which are experienced as afflictive emotion in the form of anger, hatred, desire for revenge, and so on) but rather counters their sense of injury and does not return harm for harm.

None of the foregoing is meant to imply that there are not times when it is appropriate to respond to others with strong measures. Nor does practicing patience in the sense I have described it mean that we must accept whatever people would do to us and simply give in. Nor does it mean that we should never act at all when we meet with harm. *Sö pa* should not be confused with mere passivity. On the contrary, adopting even vigorous countermeasures may be compatible with the practice of *sö pa*. There are times in everyone's life when harsh words—or even physical intervention—may be called for. But since it safeguards our inner composure, *sö pa* means we are in a stronger position to judge an appropriately non-violent response than if we are overwhelmed by negative thoughts and emotions. From this, we see that it is the very opposite of cowardice. Cowardice arises when we lose all confidence as a result of fear. Patient forbearance means that we remain firm even if we are afraid.

Nor, when I speak of acceptance, do I mean that we should not do everything in our power to solve our problems whenever they can be solved. But in the case of present suffering—that which we are already undergoing—acceptance can help ensure that the experience is not compounded by the additional burden of mental and emotional suffering. For example, there is nothing much we can do about old age. Far better to accept our condition than to fret about it. Indeed, it always strikes me as a bit foolish when elderly people proudly turn help away when obviously they need it.

Patient forbearance, then, is the quality which enables us to prevent negative thoughts and emotions from taking hold of us. It safeguards our peace of mind in the face of adversity. Through practicing patience in this way, our conduct is rendered ethically wholesome. As we have seen, the first step in ethical practice is to check our response to negative thoughts and emotions as they arise. The next step—what we do after applying the brakes—is to counter that provocation with patience.

Here the reader may object that surely there will be occasions when this is impossible. What about the times when someone we are close to, who knows all our weaknesses, behaves toward us in a way that we find ourselves unable to prevent anger from completely overwhelming our defenses? Under such circumstances, we may indeed find it impossible to preserve our compassion for the other, but at least we should take care not to react violently, or aggressively. Leaving the room and going for a walk, or even counting twenty breaths, may be the best thing: we need to find some means of calming down a bit. This is why we need to put the practice of patience at the heart of our daily lives. It is a question of familiarizing ourselves with it, at the deepest level, so that when we do find ourselves in a difficult situation, although we may have to make an extra effort, we know what is involved. On the other hand, if we ignore the practice of patience until we are actually experiencing trouble, it is quite likely we will not succeed in resisting provocation.

One of the best ways to begin familiarizing ourselves with the virtue of patience, or *sö pa,* is by taking time to reflect systematically on its benefits. It is the source of forgiveness. When *sö pa* is combined with our ability to discriminate between action and agent, forgiveness arises naturally. Moreover, *sö pa* has no equal in protecting our concern for others, whatever their behavior toward us. It enables us to reserve our judgment toward the act, and it enables us to have compassion for the individual. Similarly, when we develop the ability patiently to forebear, we find that we develop a proportionate reserve of calmness and tranquility. We tend to be less antagonistic and more pleasant to associate with. This, in turn, creates a positive atmosphere around us so that it is easy for others to relate to us. And being better grounded emotionally through the practice of patience, we find that not only do we become much stronger mentally and spiritually, but we tend also to be healthier physically. Certainly I attribute the good health I enjoy to a generally calm and peaceful mind.

But the most important benefit of *sö pa,* or patience, consists in the way it acts as a powerful antidote to the affliction of anger—the greatest threat to our inner peace, and therefore our happiness. Indeed, we find that patience is the best means we have of defending ourselves internally from anger's destructive effects. Consider: riches are no defense against anger. Nor is a person's education, no matter how accomplished and intelligent they may be. Nor, for that matter, can the law be of any help. And fame is useless. Only the inner protection of patient forbearance can keep us from experiencing the turmoil of negative thoughts and emotions. The mind, or spirit (*lo*), is not physical. It cannot be touched or harmed directly. Only negative thoughts and emotions can harm it. Therefore, only the corresponding positive quality can protect it.

As a second step to familiarizing ourselves with the virtue of patience, it is also very helpful to think of adversity not so much as a threat to our peace of mind but rather as the very means by which patience is attained. From this perspective, we see that those who would harm us are, in a sense, teachers of patience. Such people teach us what we could never learn merely from hearing someone speak, be they ever so wise or holy. No more can the reader hope to learn virtue merely by reading this book—unless, of course, it is so boring as to demand perseverance! From adversity we can, however, learn the value of patient forbearance. And, in particular, those who would harm us give us unparalleled opportunities to practice disciplined behavior.

This is not to say that people are not responsible for their actions. But let us remember that they may be acting largely out of ignorance. A child brought up in a violent environment may not know any other way to behave. As a result, the question of blame is rendered largely redundant. The appropriate response to someone who causes us to suffer—and here, of course, I am not referring to those instances when others oppose us legitimately, as when they refuse to give in to our unreasonable demands—is to recognize that in harming us, ultimately they lose their peace of mind, their inner balance, and thereby their happiness. And we do best when we have compassion for them, especially since a simple wish to see them hurt cannot actually harm them. It will certainly harm us, though.

Imagine two neighbors in dispute. One of them is able to take this dispute lightly. The other is obsessed with it and constantly schemes to find a way to hurt his or her opponent. But what happens? Nurturing malice, it is not long before the one who broods begins to suffer. First, he or she will lose their appetite, then their sleep. Eventually, their health begins to go. They pass their days and nights in misery—with the result that, ironically, they end up fulfilling the wishes of their adversary.

In fact, when we really think about it, there is something not fully rational about singling out individual persons as the objects of our anger. Let us conduct a simple exercise in our imagination. Consider the case of someone who abuses us verbally. If we feel inclined to anger on account of the pain this causes us, should not the focus of our feelings really be on the words themselves, since these are what is actually causing us pain? Yet we become angry with the individual who is shouting at us. It could, of course, be objected that since it is the person who is doing the shouting, we are justified in becoming angry with them on the grounds that we are right to assign moral responsibility to the individual and not to his or her words. This may be true. At the same time, if we are to be angry at what actually caused the pain, their words are actually the more immediate cause. Better still, should we not direct our anger toward what drove that person to abuse us: their afflictive emotions? For if the person were calm and at peace, they would not act in this way. Yet of these three factors—the words which hurt, the person uttering them, and the negative impulses which drive them—it is toward the person that we direct our anger. There is something inconsistent in this.

If it be objected that it is the nature of the one who is abusing us which is truly the cause of our pain, still we would have no reasonable grounds for anger with that individual. For if it were that person's ultimate nature to be hostile toward us, they would be incapable of behaving differently. In that case, anger toward them would be pointless. If we are burned, there is no sense in being angry with fire. It is in the nature of fire to burn. But to remind ourselves that the notion of inherent hostility or inherent evil is false, let us observe that under different circumstances, the same person who is causing us pain could become a good friend. It is not unusual to hear of soldiers on opposing sides during conflict becoming close in peacetime. And most of us have had the experience of meeting someone who despite a bad reputation in the past turns out to be quite pleasant.

Of course I am not suggesting that we should engage in such reflections as these in every situation. When we are physically threatened, we might do better to concentrate our energies not on reasoning like this but in running away! But it is helpful to spend time familiarizing ourselves with the various aspects and benefits of patience. This will enable us to meet the challenges posed by adversity in a constructive manner.

I mentioned earlier that *sö pa,* or patience, acts as a counterforce to anger. In fact, for every negative state, we find that we can identify one which opposes it. For example, humility opposes pride; contentment opposes greed; perseverance opposes indolence. If, therefore, we wish to overcome the suffering which arises when negative thoughts and emotions are allowed to develop, cultivating virtue should not be seen as separate from restraining our response to them. They go hand in hand. This is why ethical discipline cannot be confined either to mere restraint or to mere affirmation of positive qualities.

To see how this process of restraint coupled with counteraction works, let us consider anxiety. We can describe this as a form of fear, but one with a well-developed mental component. Now we are bound to encounter experiences and events we feel concerned about. But what turns concern into anxiety is when we start to brood and let the imagination add negative reflections. Then we begin to feel anxious and start to worry. And the more we indulge this, the more reasons we find for it. Eventually we may find ourselves in a state of permanent distress. The more developed this state, the less we are able to take action against it, and the stronger it becomes. But when we think carefully, we see that underlying this process is principally narrowness of vision and a lack of proper perspective. This causes us to ignore the fact that things and events come into being as the result of innumerable causes and conditions, and we tend to concentrate on just one or two aspects of our situation. For example, we attribute our suffering solely to negative childhood experiences. But in so doing, inevitably we restrict ourselves to finding means to overcoming only these aspects. The trouble with this is that if we are unable to do so, there is a danger of becoming totally demoralized. The first step in overcoming anxiety is thus to develop a proper perspective of our situation.

This we can do in a number of different ways. One of the most effective is to try to shift the focus of attention away from self and toward others. When we succeed in this, we find that the scale of our own problems diminishes. This is not to say we should ignore our own needs altogether, but rather that we should try to remember others' needs alongside our own, no matter how pressing ours may be. This is helpful, because when our concern for others is translated into action, we find that confidence arises automatically and worry and anxiety diminish. Indeed, we find that almost all the mental and emotional suffering which is such a feature of modern living—including the sense of hopelessness, of loneliness, and so on—lessens the moment we begin to engage in actions motivated by concern for others. In my opinion, this explains why merely performing outwardly positive actions will not suffice to reduce anxiety. When the underlying motive is to further one's short-term aims, we only add to our problems.

What, though, of those occasions when we find our whole lives unsatisfactory, or when we feel on the point of being overwhelmed by our suffering—as happens to us all in varying degrees from time to time? When this occurs, it is vital that we make every effort to find a way of lifting our spirits. We can do this by recollecting our good fortune. We may, for example, be loved by someone; we may have certain talents; we may have received a good education; we may have our basic needs provided for—food to eat, clothes to wear, somewhere to live—we may have performed certain altruistic deeds in the past. Not unlike a banker who collects interest even on the smallest amounts of money he has out on loan, we must take into consideration even the slightest positive aspect of our lives. For if we fail to find some way of uplifting ourselves, there is every danger of sinking further into our sense of powerlessness. This can lead us to believe that we have no capacity for doing good whatsoever. Thus we create the conditions of despair itself. At that point, suicide may seem the only option.

In most cases of hopelessness and despair, we find that it is the individual's perception of their situation rather than its reality which is the issue. Certainly, it may not be resolvable without others' co-operation. In that case, it becomes a matter of asking for help. However, there may indeed be some circumstances which are hopeless. This is where religious belief can be a source of comfort, but that is a separate matter.

What else might an ethic of virtue consist in? As a general principle, it is essential to avoid extremes. Just as overeating is as dangerous as undereating, so it is with the pursuit and practice of virtue. We find that even noble causes when carried to extremes can become a source of harm. For example, courage taken to excess and without due regard for circumstances quickly becomes foolhardiness. Indeed, excess undermines one of the principal purposes of practicing virtue, which is to offset our tendency to drastic mental and emotional reactions to others and to those events which cause us unavoidable suffering.

It is also important to realize that transforming the mind and heart so that our actions become spontaneously ethical requires that we put the pursuit of virtue at the heart of our daily lives. This is because love and compassion, patience, generosity, humility, and so on are all complementary. And because it is so difficult to eradicate afflictive emotion, it is necessary that we habituate ourselves to their opposites even before negative thoughts and emotions arise. For example, the cultivation of generosity is essential to counteract our tendency to guard our possessions and even our energy too closely. The practice of giving helps us to overcome our habit of miserliness, which we tend to justify by asking, "What will I have for myself if I start giving things away?"

Giving is recognized as a virtue in every major religion and in every civilized society, and it clearly benefits both the giver and the receiver. The one who receives is relieved from the pangs of want. The one who gives can take comfort from the joy their gift brings to others. At the same time, we must recognize that there are different types and degrees of giving. When we give with the underlying motive of inflating the image others have of us—to gain renown and have them think of us as virtuous or holy—we defile the act. In that case, what we are practicing is not generosity but self-aggrandizement. Similarly, the one who gives much may not be so generous as the one who gives little. It all depends on the giver's means and motivation.

Though not a substitute, giving of our time and energy may represent a somewhat higher order of giving than making gifts. Here I am thinking especially of the gift of service to those with mental or physical disabilities, to the homeless, to those who are lonely, to those in prison and those who have been in prison. But this type of giving also includes, for example, teachers who impart their knowledge to students. Then, as I understand it, the most compassionate form of giving is when it is done without any thought or expectation of reward, and grounded in genuine concern for others. This is because the more we can expand our focus to include others' interests alongside our own, the more securely we build the foundations of our own happiness.

To say that humility is an essential ingredient in our pursuit of transformation may seem to be at odds with what I have said about the need for confidence. But just as there is clearly a distinction between valid confidence, in the sense of self-esteem, and conceit—which we can describe as an inflated sense of importance grounded in a false image of self—so it is important to distinguish between genuine humility, which is a species of modesty, and a lack of confidence. They are not the same thing at all, though many confuse them. This may explain, in part, why today humility is often thought of as a weakness rather than as an indication of inner strength—especially in the context of business and professional life. Certainly, modern society does not accord humility the place it had in Tibet when I was young. Then, both our culture and peoples' basic admiration of humility provided a climate in which it flourished, while ambition (to be differentiated from the entirely appropriate aspiration to succeed in wholesome tasks) was seen as a quality which leads all too easily to self-centered thinking. Yet in contemporary life, humility is more important than ever. The more successful we humans become, both as individuals and as a family through our development of science and technology, the more essential it becomes to preserve humility. For the greater our temporal achievements, the more vulnerable we become to pride and arrogance.

One technique helpful in developing real confidence and humility is to reflect on the example of those whose self-importance makes them an object of ridicule to others. They may not be aware of how foolish they look, but it is plain to everyone else. This is not a matter of sitting in judgment on others, however. Rather it is a question of bringing home to ourselves the negative consequences of such states of heart and mind. By seeing, through the example of others, where they lead, we will be all the more determined to avoid them. In a sense, we are reversing the principle of not harming others on the basis that we ourselves do not wish to be harmed and making use of the fact that it is much easier to identify others' failings than it is to acknowledge their virtues. It is also much easier to find fault with others than with ourselves.

Here I should perhaps add that if humility is not to be confused with lack of confidence, still less has it anything to do with a sense of worthlessness. Lack of a proper recognition of one's own value is always harmful and can lead to a state of mental, emotional, and spiritual paralysis. Under such circumstances, the individual may even come to hate themselves, although I must admit that the concept of self-hatred seemed incoherent when it was first explained to me by some Western psychologists. It seemed to contradict the principle that our fundamental desire is to be happy and to avoid suffering. But I do now accept that when a person loses all sense of perspective, there is a danger of self-hatred. Yet we all have the capacity for empathy. We all, therefore, have the potential to engage in wholesome conduct even if this only takes the form of positive thoughts. To suppose ourselves worthless is simply incorrect.

Another way to avoid the narrowing of vision that can lead to such extreme states as self-hatred and despair is to rejoice in others' good fortune, where we find it. As part of this practice, it is helpful to take every opportunity to show our respect for others, even to encourage them with praise when that seems appropriate. If such praise seems likely to come across as flattery or to make them feel conceited, it may, of course, be better to keep our goodwill private. And when it is we ourselves who are being praised, it is vital not to let this make us feel puffed up and important. Instead, let us merely recognize the other's generosity in appreciating our good qualities.

As a means of overcoming those negative feelings toward ourselves, which arise in connection with those occasions in the past when we have neglected others' feelings and indulged our own selfish desires and interests at their expense, it is very helpful to develop an attitude of regret and repentance. Here, though, the reader should not suppose that I am advocating that sense of guilt which so many of my Western friends speak of. We do not seem to have a word in Tibetan which could translate the word "guilt" exactly. And because of its strong cultural associations, I am not certain that I have understood the concept to its fullest extent. But it seems to me that while it is natural and to be expected that we should have feelings of discomfort in relation to our past misdeeds, there is sometimes an element of self-indulgence when this is extended to feelings of guilt. It makes no sense to brood anxiously on the harmful actions we have committed in the past to the point where we become paralyzed. They are done, it is over. If the person is a believer in God, the appropriate action is to find some means of reconciliation with Him. So far as Buddhist practice is concerned, there are various rites and practices for purification. When the individual has no religious beliefs, however, it is surely a matter of acknowledging and accepting any negative feelings we may have in relation to our misdeeds and developing a sense of sorrow and regret for them. But then, rather than stopping at mere sorrow and regret, it is important to use this as the basis for resolve, for a deep-seated commitment never again to harm others and to direct our actions all the more determinedly to the benefit of others. The act of disclosure, or confession, of our negative actions to another—especially to someone we really respect and trust—will be found to be very helpful in this. Above all, we should remember that as long as we retain the capacity of concern for others, the potential for transformation remains. We are quite wrong if we merely acknowledge the gravity of our actions inwardly and then, instead of confronting our feelings, give up all hope and do nothing. This only compounds the error.

We have a saying in Tibet that engaging in the practice of virtue is as hard as driving a donkey uphill, whereas engaging in destructive activities is as easy as rolling boulders downhill. It is also said that negative impulses arise as spontaneously as rain and gather momentum just like water following the course of gravity. What makes matters worse is our tendency to indulge negative thoughts and emotions even while agreeing that we should not. It is essential, therefore, to address directly our tendency to put things off and while away our time in meaningless activities and shrink from the challenge of transforming our habits on the grounds that it is too great a task. In particular, it is important not to allow ourselves to be put off by the magnitude of others' suffering. The misery of millions is not a cause for pity. Rather it is a cause for developing compassion.

We must also recognize that the failure to act when it is clear that action is required may itself be a negative action. Where inaction is due to anger or malice or envy, afflictive emotion can be clearly cited as the motivating factor. This is as true of simple things as it is of more complex situations. If a husband does not warn his wife that a plate she is about to pick up is hot because he desires her to be burned, clearly afflictive emotion is likely to be present. On the other hand, where inaction is simply the result of indolence, the mental and emotional state of the individual may not be so gravely negative. But the consequence may still be very serious, although such inaction is attributable less to negative thoughts and emotions as to a lack of compassion. It is thus important that we are no less determined to overcome our habitual tendency to laziness than we are to exercise restraint in response to afflictive emotion.

This is no easy task, and those who are religiously minded must understand that there is no blessing or initiation—which, if only we could receive it—or any mysterious or magical formula or mantra or ritual—if only we could discover it—that can enable us to achieve transformation instantly. It comes little by little, just as a building is constructed brick by brick or, as the Tibetan expression has it, an ocean is formed drop by drop. Also, because, unlike our bodies which soon get sick, old, and worn out, the afflictive emotions never age, it is important to realize that dealing with them is a lifelong struggle. Nor should the reader suppose that what we are talking about here is the mere acquisition of knowledge. It is not even a question of developing the conviction that may come from such knowledge. What we are talking about is gaining an experience of virtue through constant practice and familiarization so that it becomes spontaneous. What we find is that the more we develop concern for others' well-being, the easier it becomes to act in others' interests. As we become habituated to the effort required, so the struggle to sustain it lessens. Eventually, it will become second nature. But there are no shortcuts.

Engaging in virtuous activities is a bit like bringing up a young child. A great many factors are involved. And, especially at the beginning, we need to be prudent and skillful in our endeavors to transform our habits and dispositions. We also need to be realistic about what we can expect to achieve. It took us a long time to become the way we are, and habits are not changed overnight. So while it is good to raise our sights as we progress, it is a mistake to judge our behavior by using the ideal as a standard, just as in college it would be foolish to judge our child's performance as a first-year student from the perspective of a graduate. Graduation is the ideal, not the standard. For this reason, far more effective than short bursts of heroic effort followed by periods of laxity is to work steadily like a stream flowing toward our goal of transformation.

One method that is very helpful in sustaining us in this life-long task of transformation is to adopt a daily routine which can be adjusted according to our progress. Of course, as with the practice of virtue in general, this is something religious practice encourages. But that is no reason why non-believers should not use some of the ideas and techniques which have served humanity so well over the course of millennia. Making a habit of concern for others' well-being, and spending a few minutes on waking in the morning reflecting on the value of conducting our lives in an ethically disciplined manner, is a good way to start the day no matter what our beliefs or lack of them. The same is true of taking some time at the end of each day to review how successful in this we have been. Such a discipline is very helpful in developing our determination not to behave self-indulgently.

If these suggestions sound somewhat onerous to the reader searching not for *nirvana* or salvation but simply for human happiness, it is worth reminding ourselves that what brings us the greatest joy and satisfaction in life are those actions we undertake out of concern for others. Indeed, we can go further. For whereas the fundamental questions of human existence, such as why we are here, where we are going, and whether the universe had a beginning, have each elicited different responses in different philosophical traditions, it is self-evident that a generous heart and wholesome actions lead to greater peace. And it is equally clear that their negative counterparts bring undesirable consequences. Happiness arises from virtuous causes. If we truly desire to be happy, there is no other way to proceed but by way of virtue: it is the method by which happiness is achieved. And, we might add, that the basis of virtue, its ground, is ethical discipline.

Chapter Eight

THE ETHIC OF COMPASSION

WE NOTED EARLIER THAT ALL THE world's major religions stress the importance of cultivating love and compassion. In the Buddhist philosophical tradition, different levels of attainment are described. At a basic level, compassion (*nying je*) is understood mainly in terms of empathy—our ability to enter into and, to some extent, share others' suffering. But Buddhists—and perhaps others—believe that this can be developed to such a degree that not only does our compassion arise without any effort, but it is unconditional, undifferentiated, and universal in scope. A feeling of intimacy toward all other sentient beings, including of course those who would harm us, is generated, which is likened in the literature to the love a mother has for her only child.

But this sense of equanimity toward all others is not seen as an end in itself. Rather, it is seen as the springboard to a love still greater. Because our capacity for empathy is innate, and because the ability to reason is also an innate faculty, compassion shares the characteristics of consciousness itself. The potential we have to develop it is therefore stable and continuous. It is not a resource which can be used up—as water is used up when we boil it. And though it can be described in terms of activity, it is not like a physical activity which we train for, like jumping, where once we reach a certain height we can go no further. On the contrary, when we enhance our sensitivity toward others' suffering through deliberately opening ourselves up to it, it is believed that we can gradually extend out compassion to the point where the individual feels so moved by even the subtlest suffering of others that they come to have an overwhelming sense of responsibility toward those others. This causes the one who is compassionate to dedicate themselves entirely to helping others overcome both their suffering and the causes of their suffering. In Tibetan, this ultimate level of attainment is called *nying je chenmo*, literally "great compassion."

Now I am not suggesting that each individual must attain these advanced states of spiritual development in order to lead an ethically wholesome life. I have described *nying je chenmo* not because it is a precondition of ethical conduct but rather because I believe that pushing the logic of compassion to the highest level can act as a powerful inspiration. If we can just keep the aspiration to develop *nying je chenmo*, or great compassion, as an ideal, it will naturally have a significant impact on our outlook. Based on the simple recognition that, just as I do, so do all others desire to be happy and not to suffer, it will serve as a constant reminder against selfishness and partiality. It will remind us that if we reserve ethical conduct for those whom we feel close to, the danger is that we will neglect our responsibilities toward those outside this circle. It will remind us that there is little to be gained from being kind and generous because we hope to win something in return. It will remind us that actions motivated by the desire to create a good name for ourselves are still selfish, however much they may appear to be acts of kindness. It will also remind us that there is nothing exceptional about acts of charity toward those we already feel close to. And it will help us to recognize that the bias we naturally feel toward our families and friends is actually a highly unreliable thing on which to base ethical conduct.

Why is this? So long as the individuals in question continue to meet our expectations, all is well. But should they fail to do so, someone we consider a dear friend one day can become our sworn enemy the next. As we saw earlier, we have a tendency to react badly to all who threaten fulfillment of our cherished desires, though they may be our closest relations. For this reason, compassion and mutual respect offer a much more solid basis for our relations with others. This is also true of partnerships. Likewise, if our love for someone is based largely on attraction, whether it be their looks or some other superficial characteristic, our feelings for that person are liable, over time, to evaporate. When they lose the quality we found alluring, or when we find ourselves no longer satisfied by it, the situation can change completely, this despite their being the same person. This is why relationships based purely on attraction are almost always unstable. On the other hand, when we begin to perfect our compassion, neither the other's appearance nor their behavior affects our underlying attitude.

Consider, too, that habitually our feelings toward others depend very much on their circumstances. Most people, when they see someone who is handicapped, feel sympathetic toward that person. But then when they see others who are wealthier, or better educated, or better placed socially, they immediately feel envious and competitive toward them. Our negative feelings prevent us from seeing the sameness of ourselves and all others. We forget that just like us, whether fortunate or unfortunate, distant or near, they desire to be happy and not to suffer.

The struggle is thus to overcome these feelings of partiality. Certainly, developing genuine compassion for our loved ones is the obvious and appropriate place to start. The impact our actions have on our close ones will generally be much greater than on others, and therefore our responsibilities toward them are greater. Yet we need to recognize that, ultimately, there are no grounds for discriminating in their favor. In this sense, we are all in the same position as a doctor confronted by ten patients suffering the same serious illness. They are each equally deserving of treatment. The reader should not suppose that what is being advocated here is a state of detached indifference, however. The further essential challenge, as we begin to extend our compassion toward all others, is to maintain the same level of intimacy as we feel toward those closest to us. In other words, what is being suggested is that we need to strive for even-handedness in our approach toward all others, a level ground into which we can plant the seed of *nying je chenmo,* of great love and compassion.

If we can begin to relate to others on the basis of such equanimity, our compassion will not depend on the fact that so and so is my husband, my wife, my relative, my friend. Rather, a feeling of closeness toward all others can be developed based on the simple recognition that, just like myself, all wish to be happy and to avoid suffering. In other words, we will start to relate to others on the basis of their sentient nature. Again, we can think of this in terms of an ideal, one which it is immensely difficult to attain. But, for myself, I find it one which is profoundly inspiring and helpful.

Let us now consider the role of compassionate love and kind-heartedness in our daily lives. Does the ideal of developing it to the point where it is unconditional mean that we must abandon our own interests entirely? Not at all. In fact, it is the best way of serving them— indeed, it could even be said to constitute the wisest course for fulfilling self-interest. For if it is correct that those qualities such as love, patience, tolerance, and forgiveness are what happiness consists in, and if it is also correct that *nying je,* or compassion, as I have defined it, is both the source and the fruit of these qualities, then the more we are compassionate, the more we provide for our own happiness. Thus, any idea that concern for others, though a noble quality, is a matter for our private lives only, is simply short-sighted. Compassion belongs to every sphere of activity, including, of course, the workplace.

Here, though, I must acknowledge the existence of a perception—shared by many, it seems—that compassion is, if not actually an impediment, at least irrelevant to professional life. Personally, I would argue that not only is it relevant, but that when compassion is lacking, our activities are in danger of becoming destructive. This is because when we ignore the question of the impact our actions have on others' well-being, inevitably we end up hurting them. The ethic of compassion helps provide the necessary foundation and motivation for both restraint and the cultivation of virtue. When we begin to develop a genuine appreciation of the value of compassion, our outlook on others begins automatically to change. This alone can serve as a powerful influence on the conduct of our lives. When, for example, the temptation to deceive others arises, our compassion for them will prevent us from entertaining the idea. And when we realize that our work itself is in danger of being exploited to the detriment of others, compassion will cause us to disengage from it. So to take an imaginary case of a scientist whose research seems likely to be a source of suffering, they will recognize this and act accordingly, even if this means abandoning the project.

I do not deny that genuine problems can arise when we dedicate ourselves to the ideal of compassion. In the case of a scientist who felt unable to continue in the direction their work was taking them, this could have profound consequences both for themselves and for their families. Likewise, those engaged in the caring professions—in medicine, counseling, social work, and so on—or even those looking after someone at home may sometimes become so exhausted by their duties that they feel over- whelmed. Constant exposure to suffering, coupled occasionally with a feeling of being taken for granted, can induce feelings of help- lessness and even despair. Or it can happen that individuals may find themselves per- forming outwardly generous actions merely for the sake of it—simply going through the motions, as it were. Of course this is better than nothing. But when left unchecked, this can lead to insensitivity toward others' suffering. If this starts to happen, it is best to disengage for a short while and make a deliberate effort to reawaken that sensitivity. In this it can be helpful to remember that despair is never a solution. It is, rather, the ultimate failure. Therefore, as the Tibetan expression has it, even if the rope breaks nine times, we must splice it back together a tenth time. In this way, even if ultimately we do fail, at least there will be no feelings of regret. And when we combine this insight with a clear appreciation of our potential to benefit others, we find that we can begin to restore our hope and confidence.

Some people may object to this ideal on the grounds that by entering into others' suffering, we bring suffering on ourselves. To an extent, this is true. But I suggest that there is an important qualitative distinction to be made between experiencing one's own suffering and experiencing suffering in the course of sharing in others'. In the case of one's own suffering, given that it is involuntary, there is a sense of oppression: it seems to come from outside us. By contrast, sharing in someone else's suffering must at some level involve a degree of voluntariness, which itself is indicative of a certain inner strength. For this reason, the disturbance it may cause is considerably less likely to paralyze us than our own suffering.

Of course, even as an ideal, the notion of developing unconditional compassion is daunting. Most people, including myself, must struggle even to reach the point where putting others' interests on a par with our own becomes easy. We should not allow this to put us off, however. And while undoubtedly there will be obstacles on the way to developing a genuinely warm heart, there is the deep consolation of knowing that in doing so we are creating the conditions for our own happiness. As I mentioned earlier, the more we truly desire to benefit others, the greater the strength and confidence we develop and the greater the peace and happiness we experience. If this still seems unlikely, it is worth asking ourselves how else we are to do so. With violence and aggression? Of course not. With money? Perhaps up to a point, but no further. But with love, by sharing in others' suffering, by recognizing ourselves clearly in all others—especially those who are disadvantaged and those whose rights are not respected—by helping them to be happy: yes. Through love, through kindness, through compassion we establish understanding between ourselves and others. This is how we forge unity and harmony.

Compassion and love are not mere luxuries. As the source both of inner and external peace, they are fundamental to the continued survival of our species. On the one hand, they constitute non-violence in action. On the other, they are the source of all spiritual qualities: of forgiveness, tolerance, and all the virtues. Moreover, they are the very thing that gives meaning to our activities and makes them constructive. There is nothing amazing about being highly educated; there is nothing amazing about being rich. Only when the individual has a warm heart do these attributes become worthwhile.

So to those who say that the Dalai Lama is being unrealistic in advocating this ideal of unconditional love, I urge them to experiment with it nonetheless. They will discover that when we reach beyond the confines of narrow self-interest, our hearts become filled with strength. Peace and joy become our constant companion. It breaks down barriers of every kind and in the end destroys the notion of my interest as independent from others' interest. But most important, so far as ethics is concerned, where love of one's neighbor, affection, kindness, and compassion live, we find that ethical conduct is automatic. Ethically wholesome actions arise naturally in the context of compassion.

Chapter Nine

ETHICS AND SUFFERING

⤟⤞ I HAVE SUGGESTED THAT WE ALL DESIRE happiness, that genuine happiness is characterized by peace, that peace is most surely attained when our actions are motivated by concern for others, and that this, in turn, entails ethical discipline and dealing positively with afflictive emotion. I have also suggested that in our quest for happiness we naturally and properly seek to avoid suffering. Let us now examine this quality, or state, that we wish so strongly to be free from but which lies at the very heart of our existence.

Suffering and pain are inalienable facts of life. A sentient being, according to my usual definition, is one which has the capacity to experience pain and suffering. One could also say that it is our experience of suffering which connects us to others. It is the basis of our capacity for empathy. But beyond this, we can observe that suffering falls into two (interrelated) categories. There are the avoidable forms which arise as a consequence of such phenomena as war, poverty, violence, crime—even things like illiteracy and certain diseases. Then there are the unavoidable forms which include such phenomena as the problems of sickness, old age, and death. So far, we have mainly been speaking about dealing with avoidable, human-created suffering. Now I want to look more closely at that which is unavoidable.

The problems and difficulties we face in life are not all like natural disasters. We cannot protect ourselves from them merely by taking suitable precautions, such as by storing food. In the case of sickness, for example, no matter how fit we keep ourselves or how carefully we regulate our diet, eventually our bodies give in to physical problems. And when they do, the impact on our lives can be serious: we may be prevented from doing the things we want to do and from going to the places we want to go. Often we are prevented from eating the foods we like. Instead, we have to take medicines which taste awful. When things get really bad, we can find ourselves enduring days and nights wracked with pain—to the extent that we may long to die.

So far as aging is concerned, from the day we are born, we are faced with the prospect of growing old and losing the suppleness of youth. In time, our hair falls out, our teeth fall out, we lose our eyesight and our hearing. We can no longer digest the foods we once enjoyed. Eventually, we find that we cannot recall events which once were so vivid, or even remember the names of those closest to us. Should we live long enough, we will reach such a state of decrepitude that others may find the mere sight of us repulsive, though that is precisely the time we will have most need of them.

Then comes death—almost a taboo subject in modern society, it seems. Though eventually we may look forward to it as a relief and regardless of what may come afterwards, death means that we are parted from our loved ones, from our precious belongings, indeed from all that we hold dear.

To this brief description of unavoidable suffering we must, however, add another category. This is the suffering entailed in meeting with the unwanted—of mishaps and accident. This is the suffering of having what we want taken away from us—as we refugees have lost our countries, many forcibly parted from their loved ones. This is the suffering caused by not obtaining what we desire, though we may put great effort into doing so. Despite breaking our back working in the fields, the harvest fails; despite working night and day at a business venture, it is not successful, though through no fault of our own. It includes also suffering uncertainty, of never knowing when and where we will meet with adversity. From our own experience, we all know how this can lead to feelings of insecurity and anxiety. And undermining everything we do, there is the suffering of lack of contentment, which arises even when we achieve all that we have striven for. Such events are part of our everyday experience as human beings who desire happiness and not to suffer.

As if this were not enough, there is furthermore the fact that the very experiences which ordinarily we suppose to be pleasurable turn out themselves to be a source of suffering. They seem to offer fulfillment, but they do not actually provide it, a phenomenon we looked at earlier in the discussion on happiness. In fact, if we think carefully, we will find that we perceive such experiences as pleasurable only insofar as they offset more explicit suffering, as when, for example, we eat to assuage hunger. We take one mouthful, then two, three, four, five, and enjoy the experience—but quite soon, although it is the same person and the same food, we begin to find eating objectionable. If we do not stop, eventually it will harm us—just as practically every worldly pleasure comes to harm us when carried to an extreme. This is why contentment is indispensable if we are to be genuinely happy.

All these manifestations of suffering are essentially unavoidable and indeed natural facts of existence. This does not mean that, finally, there is nothing we can do about them. Nor do I mean to suggest that it is unrelated to the question of ethical discipline. It is true that, according to Buddhist and other ancient Indian religious philosophies, suffering is seen as a consequence of *karma*. To suppose, as do quite a lot of people, Easterners and Westerners alike it seems, that this means that everything we experience is predetermined is totally wrong, however. Still less is it an excuse not to take responsibility in whatever situation we find ourselves.

Since the term *karma* appears to have

entered everyday vocabulary, it might be worthwhile to clarify the concept somewhat. *Karma* is a Sanskrit word meaning "action." It denotes an active force, the inference being that the outcome of future events can be influenced by our actions. To suppose that *karma* is some sort of independent energy which predestines the course of our whole life is simply incorrect. Who creates *karma*? We ourselves. What we think, say, do, desire, and omit creates *karma*. As I write, for example, the very action creates new circumstances and causes some other event. My words cause a response in the reader's mind. In everything we do, there is cause and effect, cause and effect. In our daily lives the food we eat, the work we undertake, our relaxation are all a function of action: our action. This is *karma*. We cannot, therefore, throw up our hands whenever we find ourselves confronted by unavoidable suffering. To say that every misfortune is simply the result of *karma* is tantamount to saying that we are totally powerless in life. If this were correct, there would be no cause for hope. We might as well pray for the end of the world.

A proper appreciation of cause and effect suggests that far from being powerless, there is much we can do to influence our experience of suffering. Old age, sickness, and death are inevitable. But, as with the torments of negative thoughts and emotions, we certainly have a choice in how we respond to the occurrence of suffering. If we wish, we can adopt a more dispassionate and rational approach, and on that basis we can discipline our response to it. On the other hand, we can simply fret about our misfortunes. But when we do, we become frustrated. As a result, afflictive emotions arise and our peace of mind is destroyed. When we do not restrain our tendency to react negatively to suffering, it becomes a source of negative thoughts and emotions. There is thus a clear relationship between the impact suffering has on our heart and mind and our practice of inner discipline.

Our basic attitude toward suffering makes a great difference to the way in which we experience it. Imagine, for example, two people suffering an identical form of terminal cancer. The only difference between these two patients is their outlook on it. One sees it as something to be accepted and, if possible, transformed into an opportunity for developing inner strength. The other reacts to his or her circumstances with fear, bitterness, and anxiety about the future. Now although purely in terms of physical symptoms there may be no difference between the two of them in terms of what they are suffering, in actual fact there is a profound difference in their experience of this illness. In the case of the latter, in addition to the physical suffering itself, there is the added pain of inner suffering.

This suggests that the degree to which suffering affects us is largely up to us. It is, therefore, essential to keep a proper perspective on our experience of suffering. We find that when we look at a particular problem from close up, it tends to fill our whole field of vision and look enormous. If, however, we look at the same problem from a distance, automatically we will start to see it in relation to other things. This simple act makes a tremendous difference. It enables us to see that though a given situation may truly be tragic, even the most unfortunate event has innumerable aspects and can be approached from many different angles. Indeed, it is very rare, if not impossible, to find a situation which is negative no matter how we look at it.

When tragedy or misfortune come our way, as surely they must, it can be very helpful to make a comparison with another event, or to call to mind a similar or worse situation that has befallen, if not ourselves, then others before us. If we can actually shift our focus away from self and toward others, we experience a freeing effect. There is something about the dynamics of self-absorption, or worrying about ourselves too much, which tends to magnify our suffering. Conversely, when we come to see it in relation to others' suffering, we begin to recognize that, relatively speaking, it is not all that unbearable. This enables us to maintain our peace of mind much more easily than if we concentrate on our problems to the exclusion of all else.

As far as my own experience is concerned, I find that when, for example, I hear bad news from Tibet—and sadly this is quite often—naturally my immediate response is one of great sadness. However, by placing it in context and by reminding myself that the basic human disposition toward affection, freedom, truth, and justice must eventually prevail, I find I can cope reasonably well. Feelings of helpless anger, which do nothing but poison the mind, embitter the heart, and enfeeble the will seldom arise, even following the worst news.

It is also worth remembering that the time of greatest gain in terms of wisdom and inner strength is often that of greatest difficulty. With the right approach—and here we see once more the supreme importance of developing a positive attitude—the experience of suffering can open our eyes to reality. For example, my own experience of life as a refugee has helped me realize that the endless protocol, which was such an important part of my life in Tibet, was quite unnecessary. We also find that our confidence and self-reliance can grow and our courage become strengthened as a result of suffering. This can be inferred from what we see in the world around us. Within our own refugee community, for example, among the survivors of our early years in exile are a number who, though they suffered terribly, are among the strongest spiritually—and the most cheerfully carefree individuals—I have the privilege to know. Conversely, we find that in the face of even relatively slight adversity, some people who have everything are inclined to lose hope and become despondent. There is a natural tendency for wealth to spoil us. The result is that we find it progressively more difficult to bear easily the problems everyone must encounter from time to time.

Let us now consider what options are open to us when we actually encounter a particular problem. At one extreme, we can allow ourselves to be overwhelmed. At the other, we can simply go on a picnic or take a holiday and ignore it. The third possibility is to face up to the situation directly. This involves examining it, analyzing it, determining its causes, and finding out how to deal with them.

Though this third course may occasion us additional pain in the short term, it is clearly preferable to the other two courses of action. If we try to avoid or deny a given problem by simply ignoring it or taking to drink or drugs, or even some forms of meditation or prayer as a means of escape, while there is a chance of short-term relief, the problem itself remains. Such an approach is simply avoiding the issue, not resolving it. Once again, the danger is that in addition to the initial problem, there will follow mental and emotional unrest. The afflictions of anxiety, fear, and doubt build up. Eventually, this can lead to anger and despair, with all the further potential for suffering (both for self and others) which that entails.

Imagine a disaster such as being shot in the stomach. The pain is excruciating. What are we to do? Of course, we need to have the bullet removed and we undergo surgery. This adds to the trauma. Yet we gladly accept this in order to overcome the original problem. Similarly, due to infection, or to catastrophic damage, it may be necessary to lose a limb in order to save our life. But again, naturally, we are prepared to accept this lesser form of suffering if it will spare us the greater suffering of death. It is only common sense voluntarily to undergo hardship when we see that by doing so we are able to avoid worse. Saying this, I admit that this is not always an easy judgment to make. When I was around six or seven years of age, I was inoculated against smallpox. Had I realized how much it would hurt, I doubt whether I could have been persuaded that vaccination constituted a lesser suffering than the disease itself. The pain lasted fully ten days and I still have four large scars as a result!

If the prospect of confronting our suffering head-on can sometimes seem a bit daunting, it is very helpful to remember that nothing within the realm of what we commonly experience is permanent. All phenomena are subject to change and decay. Also, as the description of reality I gave earlier suggests, we are mistaken if we ever suppose that our experience of suffering—or happiness, for that matter—can be attributed to a single source. According to the theory of dependent origination, everything that arises does so within the context of innumerable causes and conditions. If this was not so, as soon as we came into contact with something that we considered good, automatically we would become happy; whenever we came into contact with something we considered bad, automatically we would become sad. The causes of joy and sorrow would be easy to identify and life would be very simple. We would have good reason to become attached to one sort of person or thing or event and to be angry with and want to avoid others. But that is not reality.

Personally, I find enormously helpful the advice given about suffering by the great Indian scholar-saint, Shantideva. It is essential, he said, that when we face difficulties of whatever sort we do not let them paralyze us. If we do, we are in danger of being totally overwhelmed by them. Instead, using our critical faculties, we should examine the nature of the problem itself. If we find that there exists the possibility we could solve it by some means or other, there is no need for anxiety. The rational thing would then be to devote all one's energy to finding that means and acting on it. If, on the other hand, we find that the nature of the problem admits to no solution, there is no point worrying about it. If nothing can change the situation, worrying only makes it worse. Taken out of context of the philosophical text in which it appears as the culmination of a complex series of reflections, Shantideva's approach may sound somewhat simplistic. But its very beauty lies in this quality of simplicity. And no one could argue with its sheer common sense.

As to the possibility that suffering has some actual purpose, we will not go into that here.

But to the extent that our experience of suffering reminds us of what all others also endure, it serves as a powerful injunction to practice compassion and refrain from causing others pain. And to the extent that suffering awakens our empathy and causes us to connect with others, it can serve as the basis of compassion and love. Here I am reminded of the example of a great Tibetan scholar and religious practitioner who spent more than twenty years in prison enduring the most terrible treatment including torture, following the occupation of our country. During that time, those students of his who had escaped into exile would often tell me that the letters he wrote and had smuggled out of jail contained the most profound teachings on love and compassion they had ever encountered. Unfortunate events, though potentially a source of anger and despair, have equal potential to be a source of spiritual growth. Whether or not this is the outcome depends on our response.

Chapter Ten

The Need for Discernment

In our survey of ethics and spiritual development, we have spoken a great deal about the need for discipline. This may seem somewhat old-fashioned, even implausible, in an age and culture where so much emphasis is placed on the goal of self-fulfillment. But the reason for people's negative view of discipline is, I suggest, mainly due to what is generally understood by the term. People tend to associate discipline with something imposed against their will. It is worth repeating, therefore, that what we are talking about when we speak of ethical discipline is something that we adopt voluntarily on the basis of full recognition of its benefits. This is not an alien concept. We do not hesitate to accept discipline when it comes to our physical health. On doctors' advice, we avoid foods that are harmful even when we crave them. Instead, we eat those that benefit us. And while it is true that at the initial stage, self-discipline, even when voluntarily adopted, may involve hardship and even a degree of struggle, this lessens over time through habituation and diligent application. It is a bit like diverting the course of a stream. First we have to dig the channel and build up its banks. Then, when the water is released into it, we may have to make adjustments here and there. But when the course is fully established, water flows in the direction we desire.

Ethical discipline is indispensable because it is the means by which we mediate between the competing claims of my right to happiness and others' equal right. Naturally, there will always be those who suppose their own happiness to be of such importance that others' pain is of no consequence. But this is short-sighted. If the reader accepts my characterization of happiness, it follows that no one truly benefits from causing harm to others. Whatever immediate advantage is gained at the expense of someone else is necessarily only temporary. In the long run, causing others hurt and disturbing their peace and happiness causes us anxiety. Because our actions have an impact both on ourselves and others, when we lack discipline, eventually anxiety arises in our mind, and deep in our heart we come to feel a sense of disquiet. Conversely, whatever hardship it entails, disciplining our response to negative thoughts and emotions will cause us fewer problems in the long run than indulging in acts of selfishness.

Nevertheless, it is worth saying again that ethical discipline entails more than just restraint. It also entails the cultivation of virtue. Love and compassion, patience, tolerance, forgiveness, and so on are essential qualities. When they are present in our lives, everything we do becomes an instrument to benefit the whole human family. Even in terms of our daily occupation—whether this is looking after children in the home, working in a factory, or serving the community as a doctor, lawyer, businessperson, or teacher—our actions contribute toward the well-being of all. And because ethical discipline is what facilitates the very qualities which give meaning and value to our existence, it is clearly something to be embraced with enthusiasm and conscious effort.

Before looking at how we apply this inner discipline to our interactions with others, it may be worth reviewing the grounds for defining ethical conduct in terms of non-harming. As we have seen, given the complex nature of reality, it is very difficult to say that a particular act or type of act is right or wrong in itself. Ethical conduct is thus not something we engage in because it is somehow right in itself. We do so because we recognize that just as I desire to be happy and to avoid suffering, so do all others. For this reason, a meaningful ethical system divorced from the question of our experience of suffering and happiness is hard to envisage.

Of course, if we want to ask all sorts of difficult questions based on metaphysics, ethical discourse can become exceedingly complicated. Yet while it is true that ethical practice cannot be reduced to a mere exercise in logic, or to simple rule-following, whichever way we look at it, in the end we are brought back to the fundamental questions of happiness and suffering. Why is happiness good and suffering bad for us? Perhaps there is no conclusive answer. But we can observe that it is in our nature to prefer the one to the other, just as it is to prefer the better over what is merely good. We simply aspire to happiness and not to suffering. If we were to go further and ask why this is so, surely the answer would have to be something like, "That's the way it is," or, for theists, "God made us that way."

So far as the ethical character of a given action

is concerned, we have seen how this is dependent on a great many factors. Time and circumstance have an important bearing on the matter. But so, too, does an individual's freedom or lack of it. A negative act can be considered more serious when the perpetrator commits the deed with full freedom as opposed to someone who is forced to act against his or her will. Similarly, given the lack of remorse this reflects, negative acts repeatedly indulged can be considered graver than an isolated act. But we must also consider the intention behind the action, as well as its content. The overriding question, however, concerns the individual's spiritual state, their overall state of heart and mind (*kun long*) in the moment of action. Because, generally speaking, this is the area over which we have the most control, it is the most significant element in determining the ethical character of our acts. As we have seen, when our intentions are polluted by selfishness, by hatred, by desire to deceive, however much our acts may have the appearance of being constructive, inevitably their impact will be negative, both for self and others.

How, though, are we to apply this principle of non-harming when confronted with an ethical dilemma? This is where our critical and imaginative powers come in. I have described these as two of our most precious resources, and suggested that possessing them is one of the things that distinguishes us from animals. We have seen how afflictive emotions destroys them. And we have seen how impor-

151

tant they are in learning to deal with suffering. As far as ethical practice is concerned, these qualities are what enable us to discriminate between temporary and long-term benefit, to determine the degree of ethical fitness of the different courses of action open to us, and to assess the likely outcome of our actions and thereby to set aside lesser goals in order to achieve greater ones. In the case of a dilemma, we need in the first instance to consider the particularity of the situation in the light of what, in the Buddhist tradition, is called the "union of skillful means and insight." "Skillful means" can be understood in terms of the efforts we make to ensure that our deeds are motivated by compassion. "Insight" refers to our critical faculties and how, in response to the different factors involved, we adjust the ideal of non-harming to the context of the situation. We could call it the faculty of wise discernment.

Employing this faculty—which is especially important when there is no appeal to religious belief—involves constantly checking our outlook and asking ourselves whether we are being broad-minded or narrow-minded. Have we taken into account the overall situation or are we considering only specifics? Is our view short-term or long-term? Are we being short-sighted or clear-eyed? Is our motive genuinely compassionate when considered in relation to the totality of all beings? Or is our compassion limited just to our families, our friends, and those we identify with closely? Just as in the practice of discovering the true nature of our thoughts and emotions, we need to think, think, think.

Of course, it will not always be possible to devote time to careful discernment. Sometimes we have to act at once. This is why our spiritual development is of such critical importance in ensuring that our actions are ethically sound. The more spontaneous our actions, the more they will tend to reflect our habits and dispositions in that moment. If these are unwholesome, our acts are bound to be destructive. At the same time, I believe it is very useful to have a set of basic ethical precepts to guide us in our daily lives. These can help us to form good habits, although I should add my opinion that in adopting such precepts, it is perhaps best to think of them less in terms of moral legislation than as reminders always to keep others' interests at heart and in the forefront of our minds.

So far as the content of such precepts is concerned, it is doubtful whether we could do better than turn to the basic ethical directives articulated not only by each of the world's great religions but also by the greater part of the humanist philosophical tradition. The consensus among them, despite differences of opinion concerning metaphysical grounding, is to my mind compelling. All agree on the negativity of killing, stealing, telling lies, and sexual misconduct. In addition, from the point of view of motivational factors, all agree on the need to avoid hatred, pride, malicious intent, covetousness, envy, greed, lust, harmful ideologies (such as racism), and so on.

Some people may wonder whether the injunctions against sexual misconduct are really necessary in these times of simple and effective contraception. However, as human beings, we are naturally attracted to external objects, whether it be through the eyes, when we are attracted by form, through the ears, when the attraction arises in relation to sound, or through any of the other senses. Each of them has the potential to be a source of difficulty for us. Yet sexual attraction involves all five senses. As a result, when extreme desire accompanies sexual attraction, it has the ability to cause us enormous problems. It is, I believe, this fact that is recognized in the ethical directives against sexual misconduct articulated by every major religion. And, at least in the Buddhist tradition, they remind us of the tendency for sexual desire to become obsessive. It can quickly reach the point where a person has almost no room left for constructive activity. In this connection, consider, for example, a case of infidelity. Given that wholesome ethical conduct entails considering the impact of our actions not only on ourselves but on others, too, there are the feelings of third parties to consider. In addition to our actions being violent toward our partner, given the trust that the relationship implies, there is the question of the lasting impact this kind of upset in the family can have on our children. It is now more or less universally accepted that they are the principal victims both of family breakup and of unhealthy relationships in the home. From our own perspective as the person who has committed the act, we must also acknowledge that it is likely to have the negative effect of gradually corroding our self-respect. Finally, there is the fact that in being unfaithful, other gravely negative acts may result as a direct consequence—lying and deception being perhaps the least of them. An unwanted pregnancy could easily be the cause of a desperate prospective parent to seeking an abortion.

When we think in this way, it becomes obvious that the momentary pleasures afforded by an adulterous liaison are far outweighed by the risk of the likely negative impact of our actions on both ourselves and others. So rather than seeing strictures against sexual misconduct as limiting to freedom, we do better to see them as commonsense reminders that such actions directly affect the well-being of both oneself and others.

Does this mean that merely following precepts takes precedence over wise discernment? No. Ethically sound conduct depends on us applying the principle of non-harming. However, there are bound to be situations when any course of action would appear to involve breaking a precept. Under such circumstances, we must use our intelligence to judge which course of action will be least harmful in the long run. Imagine, for example, a situation where we witness someone running away from a group of people armed with knives and clearly intent on doing him harm. We see the fugitive disappear into a doorway. Moments later, one of the pursuers comes up to us and asks which way he went. Now, on the one hand, we do not want to lie, to injure the other's trust. On the other, if we tell the truth, we realize that we may contribute to the injury or death of a fellow human being. Whatever we decide, the appropriate course of action would appear to involve a negative deed. Under such circumstances, because we are certain that in so doing we are serving a higher purpose—preserving someone from harm—it might well be appropriate to say, "Oh, I didn't see him" or vaguely, "I think he went the other way." We have to take into account the overall situation and weigh the benefits of telling a lie or telling the truth and do what we judge to be least harmful overall. In other words, the moral value of a given act is to be judged in relation both to time, place, and circumstance and to the interests of the totality of all others in the future as well as now. But while it is conceivable that a given act is ethically sound under one particular set of circumstances, the same act at another time and place and under a different set of circumstances may not be.

What, though, are we to do when it comes to others? What are we to do when they seem clearly to be engaging in actions which we consider wrong? The first thing is to remember that unless we know down to the last detail the full range of circumstances, both internal and external, we can never be sufficiently clear enough about individual situations to be able to judge with complete certainty the moral content of others' actions. Of course, there will be extreme situations when the negative character of others' acts will be self-evident. But mostly this is not the case. This is why it is far more useful to be aware of a single shortcoming in ourselves than it is to be aware of a thousand in somebody else. For when the fault is our own, we are in a position to correct it.

Nevertheless, remembering that there is an essential distinction to be made between a person and their particular acts, we may come across circumstances when it is appropriate to take action. In everyday life, it is normal and fitting to adapt in some degree to one's friends and acquaintances and to respect their wishes. The ability to do so is considered a good quality. But when we mix with those who clearly indulge in negative behavior, seeking only their own benefit and ignoring others', we risk losing our own sense of direction. As a result, our ability to help others becomes endangered. There is a Tibetan proverb which says that when we lie on a mountain of gold, some of it rubs off on us; the same happens if we lie on a mountain of dirt. We are right to avoid such people, though we must be careful not to cut them off completely. Indeed, there are sure to be times when it is appropriate to try to stop them from acting in this way—

provided, of course, that our motives in doing so are pure and our methods are non-harming. Again, the key principles are compassion and insight.

The same is true in respect to those ethical dilemmas we face at the level of society, especially the difficult and challenging questions posed by modern science and technology. For example, in the field of medicine, it has become possible to prolong life in cases which just a few years ago would have been hopeless. This can, of course, be a source of great joy. But quite often, there arise complicated and very delicate questions concerning the limits of care. I think that there can be no general rule in respect to this. Rather, there is likely to be a multiplicity of competing considerations, which we must assess in the light of reason and compassion. When it becomes necessary to make a difficult decision on behalf of a patient, we must take into account all the various different elements. These will, of course, be different in each case. For example, if we prolong the life of a person who is critically ill but whose mind remains lucid, we give that person the opportunity to think and feel in a way that only a human being can. On the other hand, we must consider whether in doing so they will experience great physical and mental suffering as a result of extreme measures taken to keep them alive. This in itself is not an overriding factor, however. As someone who believes in the continuation of consciousness after the death of the body, I would argue that it is much better to have pain with this human body. At least we can benefit from others' care whereas, if we choose to die, we may find that we have to endure suffering in some other form.

If the patient is not conscious and therefore unable to participate in the decision-making process, that is yet another problem. And on top of everything, there may be the wishes of the family to take into account, along with the immense problems that prolonged care can cause them and others. For example, it may be that in order to continue to support one life, valuable funds are kept from projects which would benefit many others. If there is a general principle, I think it is simply that we recognize the supreme preciousness of life and try to ensure that when the time comes, the dying person departs as serenely and peacefully as possible.

In the case of work in such fields as genetics and biotechnology, the principle of non-harming takes on special importance because lives may be at stake. When the motivation behind such research is merely profit, or fame, or even when research is carried out merely for its own sake, it is very much open to question where it will lead. I am thinking particularly of the development of techniques to manipulate physical attributes, such as gender or even hair and eye color, which can be used commercially to exploit the prejudices of parents. Indeed, let me say here that while it is difficult to be categorically against all forms of genetic experimentation, this is such a delicate area that it is essential that all those involved proceed with caution and deep humility. They must be especially aware of the potential for abuse. It is vital that they keep in mind the wider implications of what they are doing and, most important, ensure that their motives are genuinely compassionate. For if the general principle behind such work is simply utility, whereby those that are deemed useless can legitimately be used to benefit those judged to be useful, then there is nothing to stop us from subordinating the rights of those who fall into the former category to those who fall into the latter. Yet the attribute of utility can surely never justify the deprivation of an individual's rights. This is a highly dangerous and very slippery slope.

Recently I saw a BBC television documentary about cloning. Using computer-generated imagery, this film showed a creature scientists were working on, a sort of semi-human being with large eyes and several other recognizably human features lying down in a cage. Of course, at present this is just fantasy, but, they explained, it is possible to foresee a time when it will be possible to create beings like this. They could then be bred and their organs and other parts of their anatomy used in "spare parts" surgery for the benefit of human beings. I was utterly appalled at this. Oh, terrible. Surely this is taking scientific endeavor to an extreme? The idea that one day we might actually create sentient beings specifically for that purpose horrifies me. I felt the same at this prospect as I do at the idea of experiments involving human fetuses.

At the same time, it is difficult to see how this kind of thing can be prevented in the absence of individuals' disciplining their own actions. Yes, we can promulgate laws. Yes, we can have international codes of conduct—as indeed we should have both. Yet if the individual scientists do not have any sense that what they are doing is grotesque, destructive, and negative in the extreme, then there is no real prospect of putting an end to such disturbing endeavors.

What about issues like vivisection, where animals are routinely caused terrible suffering before being killed as a means to furthering scientific knowledge? Here I only want to say that to a Buddhist, such practices are equally shocking. I can only hope that the rapid advances being made in computer technology will mean there is less and less call for animal experimentation in scientific research. One positive development within modern society is the way in which, together with a growing appreciation of the importance of human rights, people are coming to have greater concern for animals. For example, there is growing recognition of the inhumanity of factory farming. It seems, too, that more and more people are taking an interest in vegetarianism and cutting down on their consumption of meat. I welcome this. My hope is that in the future, this concern will be extended to consideration for even the smallest creatures of the sea.

Here, though, I should perhaps sound a word of warning. The campaigns to protect human and animal life are noble causes. But it is essential that we do not allow ourselves to be carried away by our sense of injustice so that we ignore others' rights. We need to ensure that we are wisely discerning in pursuit of our ideals.

Exercising our critical faculties in the ethical realm entails taking responsibility both for our acts and for their underlying motives. If we do not take responsibility for our motives, whether positive or negative, the potential for harm is much greater. As we have seen, negative emotions are the source of unethical behavior. Each act affects not only the people closest to us but also our colleagues, friends, community, and, ultimately, the world.

III

ETHICS AND SOCIETY

Chapter Eleven

UNIVERSAL RESPONSIBILITY

I BELIEVE THAT OUR EVERY ACT HAS A universal dimension. Because of this, ethical discipline, wholesome conduct, and careful discernment are crucial ingredients for a meaningful, happy life. But let us now consider this proposition in relation to the wider community.

In the past, families and small communities could exist more or less independently of one another. If they took into account their neighbors' well-being, so much the better. Yet they could survive quite well without this kind of perspective. Such is no longer the case. Today's reality is so complex and, on the material level at least, so clearly interconnected that a different outlook is needed. Modern economics is a case in point. A stock-market crash on one side of the globe can have a direct effect on the economies of countries on the other. Similarly, our technological achievements are now such that our activities have an unambiguous effect on the natural environment. And the very size of our population means that we cannot any longer afford to ignore others' interests.

Indeed, we find that these are often so intertwined that serving our own interests benefits others, even though this may not be our explicit intention. For example, when two families share a single water source, ensuring that it is not polluted benefits both.

In view of this, I am convinced that it is essential that we cultivate a sense of what I call universal responsibility. This may not be an exact translation of the Tibetan term I have in mind, *chi sem*, which means, literally, universal (*chi*) consciousness (*sem*). Although the notion of responsibility is implied rather than explicit in the Tibetan, it is definitely there. When I say that on the basis of concern for others' well-being we can, and should, develop a sense of universal responsibility, I do not, however, mean to suggest that each individual has a direct responsibility for the existence of, for example, wars and famines in different parts of the world. It is true that in Buddhist practice we constantly remind ourselves of our duty to serve all sentient beings in every universe. Similarly, the theist recognizes that devotion to God entails devotion to the welfare of all His creatures. But clearly certain things, such as the poverty of a single village ten thousand miles away, are completely beyond the scope of the individual. What is entailed, therefore, is not an admission of guilt but, again, a reorientation of our heart and mind away from self and toward others. To develop a sense of universal responsibility—of the universal dimension of our every act and of the equal right of all others to happiness and not to suffer—is to develop an attitude of mind whereby, when we see an opportunity to benefit others, we will take it in preference to merely looking after our own narrow interests. But though, of course, we care about what is beyond our scope, we accept it as part of nature and concern ourselves with doing what we can.

An important benefit of developing such a sense of universal responsibility is that it helps us become sensitive to all others—not just those closest to us. We come to see the need to care especially for those members of the human family who suffer most. We recognize the need to avoid causing divisiveness among our fellow human beings. And we become aware of the overwhelming importance of contentment.

When we neglect others' well-being and ignore the universal dimension of our actions, it is inevitable that we will come to see our interests as separate from theirs. We will overlook the fundamental oneness of the human family. Of course, it is easy to point to numerous factors which work against this notion of unity. These include differences of religious faith, of language, customs, culture, and so on. But when we put too much emphasis on superficial differences, and on account of them make even small, rigid discriminations, we cannot avoid bringing about additional suffering both for ourselves and others. This makes no sense. We humans already have enough problems. We all face death, old age, and sickness—not to mention the inevitability of meeting with disappointment. These we simply cannot avoid. Is this not enough? What is the point of creating still more unnecessary problems simply on the basis of different ways of thinking or different skin color?

Judging these realities, we see that both ethics and necessity call for the same response. In order to overcome our tendency to ignore others' needs and rights, we must continually remind ourselves of what is obvious: that basically we are all the same. I come from Tibet; most of the readers of this book will not be Tibetans. If I were to meet each reader individually and look them over, I would see that the majority do indeed have characteristics superficially different from mine. If I were then to concentrate on these differences, I could certainly amplify them and make them into something important. But the result would be that we grew more distant rather than closer. If, on the other hand, I were to look on each as one of my own kind—as a human being like myself with one nose, two eyes, and so forth, ignoring differences of shape and color— then automatically that sense of distance would fade. I would see that we have the same human flesh and that, moreover, just as I want to be happy and to avoid suffering, so do they. On the basis of this recognition, I would quite naturally feel well disposed toward them. And concern for their well-being would arise almost by itself.

Yet it seems to me that while most people are willing to accept the need for unity within their own group and, within this, the need to consider others' welfare, the tendency is to neglect the rest of humanity. In doing so, we ignore not only the interdependent nature of reality but the reality of our situation. If it were possible for one group, or one race, or one nation to gain complete satisfaction and fulfillment by remaining totally independent and self-sufficient within the confines of their own society, then perhaps it could be argued that discrimination against outsiders is justifiable. But this is not the case. In fact, the modern world is such that the interests of a particular community can no longer be considered to lie within the confines of its own boundaries.

Cultivating contentment is therefore crucial to maintaining peaceful coexistence. Discontentment breeds acquisitiveness, which can never be satisfied. It is true that, if what the individual seeks is by nature infinite, such as the quality of tolerance, the question of contentment does not arise. The more we enhance our ability to be tolerant, the more tolerant we will become. In respect of spiritual qualities, contentment is neither necessary nor in fact is it desirable. But if what we seek is finite, there is every danger that having acquired it, we will still not be satisfied. In the case of the desire for wealth, even if a person were somehow able to take over the economy of an entire country, there is every chance they would begin to think in terms of acquiring that of other countries too. Desire for what is finite can never really be sated. On the other hand, when we develop contentment, we can never be disappointed or disillusioned.

Lack of contentment—which really comes down to greed—sows the seed of envy and aggressive competitiveness, and leads to a culture of excessive materialism. The negative atmosphere this creates becomes the context for all kinds of social ills which bring suffering to all members of that community. If it were the case that greed and envy had no side effects, arguably this would be a matter for that community alone. But, again, such is not the case. In particular, lack of contentment is the source of damage to our natural environment and, thereby, of harm to others. Which others? In particular, the poor and the weak. Within their own community, though the rich may be able to move to avoid, for example, high levels of pollution, the poor have no choice.

Similarly, the people of the poorer nations, which do not have the resources to cope, also suffer both from the richer nations' excesses and from the pollution of their own cruder technology. The coming generations, too, will suffer. And eventually we ourselves will suffer. How? We have to live in the world we are helping to create. If we choose not to modify our behavior out of respect for others' equal right to happiness and not to suffer, it will not be long before we begin to notice the negative consequences. Imagine the pollution of an extra two billion cars, for example. It would affect us all. So contentment is not merely an ethical matter. If we do not wish to add to our own experience of suffering, it is a matter of necessity.

This is one of the reasons why I believe that the culture of perpetual economic growth needs to be questioned. In my view, it fosters discontent, and with this comes a great number of problems, both social and environmental. There is also the fact that in devoting ourselves so wholeheartedly to material development we neglect the implications this has for the wider community. Again, this is less a matter of the gap between First and Third World, North and South, between developed and underdeveloped, between rich and poor, being immoral and wrong. It is both of these. But in some ways more significant is the fact that such inequality is itself the source of trouble for everyone. If it were the case that, for example, Europe was the whole world, rather than home to less than ten percent of the world's population, the prevailing ideology of endless growth might be justifiable. Yet the world is more than just Europe. The fact is that elsewhere people are starving. And where there are imbalances as profound as these, there are bound to be negative consequences for all, even if they are not equally direct: the rich also feel the symptoms of poverty in their daily lives. Consider, in this context, how the sight of surveillance cameras, and of iron security bars over our windows, actually detracts a little from our sense of serenity.

Universal responsibility also leads us to commitment to the principle of honesty. What do I mean by this? We can think of honesty and dishonesty in terms of the relationship between appearance and reality. Sometimes these synchronize, often they do not. But when they do, that is honesty, as I understand it. So we are honest when our actions are what they seem to be. When we pretend to be one thing but in reality we are something else, suspicion develops in others, causing fear. And fear is something we all wish to avoid. Conversely, when in our interactions with our neighbors we are open and sincere in everything we say and think and do, people have no need to fear us. This holds true both for the individual and for communities. Moreover, when we understand the value of honesty in all our undertakings, we recognize that there is no ultimate difference between the needs of the individual and the needs of whole communities. Their numbers vary, but their desire, and right, not to be deceived remains the same. Thus when we commit ourselves to honesty, we help reduce the level of misunderstanding, doubt, and fear throughout society. In a small but significant way, we create the conditions for a happy world.

The question of justice is also closely connected both with universal responsibility and the question of honesty. Justice entails a requirement to act when we become aware of injustice. Indeed, failure to do so may be wrong, although not wrong in the sense that it makes us somehow intrinsically bad. But if our hesitance to speak out comes from a sense of self-centeredness, then there may be a problem. If our response to injustice is to ask, "What will happen to me if I speak out? Maybe people won't like me," this could well be unethical because we are ignoring the wider implications of our silence. It is also inappropriate and unhelpful when set in the context of all others' equal right to happiness and to avoid suffering. This remains true even—perhaps especially—when, for example, governments or institutions say, "This is our business" or "This is an internal affair." Not only can our speaking out under such circumstances be a duty, but more importantly it can be a service to others.

It may, of course, be objected that such honesty is not always possible, that we need to be "realistic." Our circumstances may prevent us from always acting in accordance with our responsibilities. Our own families may be harmed if, for example, we speak out when we witness injustice. But while we do have to deal with the day-to-day reality of our lives, it is essential to keep a broad perspective. We must evaluate our own needs in relation to the needs of others and consider how our actions and inactions are likely to affect them in the longer term. It is hard to criticize those who fear for their loved ones. But occasionally it will be necessary to take risks in order to benefit the wider community.

A sense of responsibility toward all others also means that, both as individuals and as a society of individuals, we have a duty to care for each member of our society. This is true irrespective of their physical capacity or of their capacity for mental reflection. Just like ourselves, such people have a right to happiness and to avoid suffering. We must therefore avoid, at all cost, the urge to shut away those who are grievously afflicted as if they were a burden. The same goes for those who are diseased or marginalized. To push them away would be to heap suffering on suffering. If we ourselves were in the same condition, we would look to others for help. We need, therefore, to ensure that the sick and afflicted person never feels helpless, rejected, or unprotected. Indeed, the affection we show to such people is, in my opinion, the measure of our spiritual health, both at the level of the individual and at that of society.

I may sound hopelessly idealistic in all this talk of universal responsibility. Nevertheless, it is an idea I have been expressing publicly ever since my first visit to the West, back in 1973. In those days, many people were skeptical of such notions. Similarly, it was not always easy to interest people in the concept of world peace. I am encouraged to note that today, however, an increasing number are beginning to respond favorably to these ideas.

As a result of the many extraordinary events humanity has experienced during the course of the twentieth century, we have, I feel, become more mature. In the fifties and sixties, and in some places even more recently, many people felt that ultimately conflicts should be resolved through war. Today, that thinking holds sway only in the minds of a small minority. And whereas in the early part of this century many people believed that progress and development within society should be pursued through strict regimentation, the collapse of fascism, followed later by the disappearance of the so-called Iron Curtain, has shown this to be a hopeless enterprise. It is worth noting the lesson from history which shows that order imposed by force is only ever short-lived. Moreover, the consensus (among some Buddhists too) that science and spirituality are incompatible no longer holds so firmly. Today, as the scientific understanding of the nature of reality deepens, this perception is changing. Because of this, people are beginning to show more interest in what I have called our inner world. By this, I mean the dynamics and functions of consciousness, or spirit: our hearts and minds. There has also been a worldwide increase in environmental awareness, and a growing recognition that neither individuals nor even whole nations can solve all their problems by themselves, that we need one another. To me, these are all very encouraging developments, which are sure to have far-reaching consequences. I am also encouraged by the fact that, regardless of its implementation, there is at least clearer acknowledgment of the need to seek non-violent resolutions of conflict in a spirit of reconciliation. There is also, as we have noted, growing acceptance of the universality of human rights and indeed of the need to accept diversity in areas of common importance, such as, for example, in religious affairs. This I believe to reflect a recognition of the need for a wider perspective in response to the diversity of the human family itself. As a result, despite so much suffering continuing to be inflicted on individuals and peoples in the name of ideology, or religion, or progress, or development, or economics, a new sense of hope is emerging for the downtrodden. Although it will undoubtedly be difficult to bring about genuine peace and harmony, clearly it can be done. The potential is there. And its foundation is a sense of responsibility on the part of each of us as individuals toward all others.

Chapter Twelve

LEVELS OF COMMITMENT

THROUGH DEVELOPING AN ATTITUDE OF responsibility toward others, we can begin to create the kinder, more compassionate world we all dream of. The reader may or may not agree with my advocacy of universal responsibility. But if it is correct that, given the broadly interdependent nature of reality, our habitual distinction between self and other is in some sense an exaggeration, and if on the basis of this I am right in suggesting that our aim should be to extend our compassion toward all others, we cannot avoid the conclusion that compassion—which entails ethical conduct—belongs at the heart of all our actions, both individual and social. Furthermore, although of course the details are open to debate, I am convinced that universal responsibility means that compassion belongs in the political arena too. It tells us something important about how we are to conduct our daily lives if we desire to be happy in the way I have characterized happiness. Saying this, I trust it is clear that I am not calling on everyone to renounce their present way of life and adopt some new rule or way of thinking. Rather, my intention is to suggest that the individual, keeping his or her daily way of life, can change, can become a better, more compassionate, and happier human being. And through being better, more compassionate individuals, we can begin to implement our spiritual revolution.

The work of a person laboring in some humble occupation is no less relevant to the well-being of society than that of, for example, a doctor, a teacher, a monk, or a nun. All human endeavor is potentially great and noble. So long as we carry out our work with good motivation, thinking, "My work is for others," it will be of benefit to the wider community. But when concern for others' feelings and welfare is missing, our activities tend to become spoiled. Through lack of basic human feeling, religion, politics, economics, and so on can be rendered dirty. Instead of serving humanity, they become agents of its destruction.

Therefore, in addition to developing a sense of universal responsibility, we need actually to be responsible people. Until we put our principles into practice, they remain just that. So, for example, it is appropriate for a politician who is genuinely responsible to conduct himself or herself with honesty and integrity. It is appropriate for a businessman or woman to consider the needs of others in every enterprise they undertake. It is appropriate for a lawyer to use their expertise to fight for justice.

Of course it is difficult to articulate precisely how our behavior would be shaped by a commitment to the principle of universal responsibility. For this reason, I do not have any particular standard in mind. All that I hope is that if what is written here makes sense to you, the reader, you will strive to be compassionate in your daily life, and that out of a sense of responsibility toward all others you will do what you can to help them. When you walk past a dripping tap, you will turn it off. If you see a light burning unnecessarily, you will do the same. If you are a religious practitioner and tomorrow you meet someone of another religious tradition, you will show them the same respect as you would hope them to show you. Or if you are a scientist and you see that the research you are engaged in may cause harm to others, out of a sense of responsibility you will desist from it. According to your own resources, and recognizing the limitations of your circumstances, you will do what you can. Apart from this, I am not calling for any commitment as such. And if on some days your actions are more compassionate than on others—well, that is normal. Likewise, if what I say does not seem helpful, then no matter. The important thing is that whatever we do for others, whatever sacrifices we make, it should be voluntary and arise from understanding the benefit of such actions.

On a recent visit to New York, a friend told me that the number of billionaires in America had increased from seventeen just a few years ago to several hundred today. Yet at the same time, the poor remain poor and in some cases are becoming poorer. This I consider to be completely immoral. It is also a potential source of problems. While millions do not even have the basic necessities of life—adequate food, shelter, education, and medical facilities—the inequity of wealth distribution is a scandal. If it were the case that everyone had a sufficiency for their needs and more, then perhaps a luxurious lifestyle would be tenable. If that was what the individual really wanted, it would be difficult to argue that they need refrain from exercising their right to live as they see fit. Yet things are not like that. In this one world of ours, there are areas where people throw surplus food away while others close by—our fellow humans, innocent children among them—are reduced to scavenging among rubbish, and many starve. Thus although I cannot say that the life of luxury lead by the rich is wrong of itself, assuming they are using their own money and have not acquired it dishonestly, I do say that it is unworthy, that it is spoiling.

Moreover, it strikes me that the lifestyles of the rich are often absurdly complicated. One friend of mine who stayed with an extremely wealthy family told me that every time they went swimming, they were handed a robe to wear after. This would then be changed for a fresh one each time they used the pool, even if they did so several times in one day. Extraordinary! Ridiculous, even. I do not see how living like this adds anything to one's comfort. As human beings we have only one stomach. There is a limit to the amount we can eat. Similarly, we have only eight fingers and two thumbs, so we cannot wear a hundred rings. Whatever argument there may be concerning choice, the extra we have is of no purpose in the moment when we are actually wearing a ring. The rest lie useless in their boxes. The appropriate use of wealth, as I explained to the members of one hugely prosperous Indian family, is found in philanthropic giving. In this particular case, I suggested—since they asked—that perhaps spending their money on education would be the best thing they could do. The future of the world is in our children's hands.

Therefore, if we wish to bring about a more compassionate—and therefore fairer society—it is essential that we educate our children to be responsible, caring human beings. When a person is born rich, or acquires wealth by some other means, they have a tremendous opportunity to benefit others. What a waste when that opportunity is squandered on self-indulgence.

I feel strongly that luxurious living is inappropriate, so much so that I must admit that whenever I stay in a comfortable hotel and see others eating and drinking expensively while outside there are people who do not even have anywhere to spend the night, I feel greatly disturbed. It reinforces my feeling that I am no different from either the rich or the poor. We are the same in wanting happiness and not to suffer. And we have an equal right to that happiness. As a result, I feel that if I were to see a workers' demonstration going by, I would certainly join in. And yet, of course, the person who is saying these things is one of those enjoying the comforts of the hotel. Indeed, I must go further. It is also true that I possess several valuable wrist-watches. And while I feel that if I were to sell them I could perhaps build some huts for the poor, so far I have not. In the same way, I do feel that if I were to observe a strictly vegetarian diet not only would I be setting a better example, but I would also be helping to save innocent animals' lives. So far I have not and therefore must admit a discrepancy between my principles and my practice in certain areas. At the same time, I do not believe everyone can or should be like Mahatma Gandhi and live the life of a poor peasant. Such dedication is wonderful and greatly to be admired. But the watchword is "As much as we can"—without going to extremes.

Chapter Thirteen

ETHICS IN SOCIETY

WHEN WE ARE COMMITTED TO THE ideal of concern for all others, it follows that this should inform our social and political policies. I say this not because I suppose that thereby we will be able to solve all society's problems overnight. Rather, it is my conviction that unless this wider sense of compassion which I have been urging on the reader inspires our politics, our policies are likely to harm instead of serve humanity as a whole. We must, I believe, take practical steps to acknowledge our responsibility to all others both now and in the future. This is true even where there may be little practical difference between those policies that are motivated by this compassion and those that are motivated by, for example, national interest.

Now although it is certainly the case that if all my suggestions concerning compassion, inner discipline, wise discernment, and the cultivation of virtue were to be implemented widely, the world would automatically become a kinder, more peaceful place, I believe that reality compels us to tackle our problems at the level of society at the same time as that of the individual. The world will change when each individual makes the attempt to counter their negative thoughts and emotions and when we practice compassion for its inhabitants irrespective of whether or not we have direct relationships with them.

In view of this, there are, I believe, a number of areas to which we need to give special consideration in the light of universal responsibility. These include education, the media, our natural environment, politics and economics, peace and disarmament, and interreligious harmony. Each has a vital role to play in shaping the world we live in, and I propose to examine them briefly in turn.

Before doing so, I must stress that the views I express are personal. They are also the views of someone who claims no expertise with respect to the technicalities of these matters. But if what I say seems objectionable, my hope is that it will at least give the reader pause for thought. For although it would not be surprising to see a divergence of opinion concerning how they are to be translated into actual policies, the need for compassion, for basic spiritual values, for inner discipline and the importance of ethical conduct generally are in my view incontrovertible.

Whether visiting one of our schools for Tibetan refugees in India or speaking to student audiences abroad, I am always very happy to meet young people. They have a natural enthusiasm for justice and peace, and they tend to be much more open and flexible of mind than adults. No matter how well disposed toward change we are, we adults undoubtedly find it more difficult. Meeting the young also reminds me that children constitute humanity's most precious resource. Given that their moral outlook is largely shaped by their upbringing, it is essential we educate them responsibly.

The human mind (*lo*) is both the source and, properly directed, the solution to all our problems. Those who attain great learning but lack a good heart are in danger of falling prey to the anxieties and restlessness which result from desires incapable of fulfillment. Conversely, a genuine understanding of spiritual values has the opposite effect. When we bring up our children to have knowledge without compassion, their attitude toward others is likely to be a mixture of envy of those in positions above them, aggressive competitiveness toward their peers, and scorn for those less fortunate. This leads to a propensity toward greed, presumption, excess, and, very quickly, to loss of happiness. Knowledge is important. But much more so is the use toward which it is put. This depends on the heart and mind of the one who uses it.

Education is much more than a matter of imparting the knowledge and skills by which narrow goals are achieved. It is also about opening the child's eyes to the needs and rights of others. We must show children that their actions have a universal dimension. And we must somehow find a way to build on their natural feelings of empathy so that they come to have a sense of responsibility toward others. For it is this which stirs us into action. Indeed, if we had to choose between learning and virtue, the latter is definitely more valuable. The good heart which is the fruit of virtue is by itself a great benefit to humanity. Mere knowledge is not.

How, though, are we to teach morality to our children? I have a sense that, in general, modern educational systems neglect discussion of ethical matters. This is probably not intentional so much as a by-product of historical reality. Secular educational systems were developed at a time when religious institutions were still highly influential throughout society. Because ethical and human values were and still are generally held to fall within the scope of religion, it was assumed that this aspect of a child's education would be looked after through his or her religious upbringing. This worked well enough until the influence of religion began to decline. But now, though the need is still there, it is not being met. Therefore, we must find some other way of showing children that basic human values are important. We must also help them to develop these values.

Ultimately, of course, the importance of concern for others is learned not from words but from actions: the example we set. This is why the family environment itself is such a vital component in a child's upbringing. When a caring and compassionate atmosphere is absent from the home, when children are neglected by their parents, it is easy to recognize their damaging effects. The children tend to feel helpless and insecure, and their minds are often agitated. Conversely, when children receive constant affection and protection, they tend to be much happier and more confident in their abilities. Their physical health tends to be better too. And we find that they are concerned not just for themselves but for others as well. The home environment is also important because children learn negative behavior from their parents. If, for example, the father is always getting into fights with his associates, or if the father and mother are always arguing destructively, although at first the child may find this objectionable, eventually they will come to understand it as quite normal. This learning is then taken out of the home and into the world.

It also goes without saying that what children learn about ethical conduct at school has to be practiced first. In this, teachers have a special responsibility. By their own behavior, they can make children remember them for their whole lives. If this behavior is principled, disciplined, and compassionate, their values will be readily impressed on the child's mind. This is because the lessons taught by a teacher with a positive motivation (*kun long*) penetrate deepest into their students' minds. I know this from my own experience. As a boy, I was very lazy. But when I was aware of the affection and concern of my tutors, their lessons would generally sink in much more successfully than if one of them was harsh or unfeeling that day.

So far as the specifics of education are concerned, that is for the experts. I will, therefore, confine myself to a few suggestions. The first is that in order to awaken young people's consciousness to the importance of basic human values, it is better not to present society's problems purely as an ethical matter or as a religious matter. It is important to emphasize that what is at stake is our continued survival. This way, they will come to see that the future lies in their hands. Secondly, I do believe that dialogue can and should be taught in class. Presenting students with a controversial issue and having them debate it is a wonderful way to introduce them to the concept of resolving conflict non-violently. Indeed, one would hope that if schools were to make this a priority, it could have a beneficial effect on family life itself. On seeing his or her parents wrangling, a child that had understood the value of dialogue would instinctively say, "Oh, no. That's not the way. You have to talk, to discuss things properly."

Finally, it is essential that we eliminate from our schools' curricula any tendency toward presenting others in a negative light.

There are undoubtedly some parts of the world where the teaching of history, for example, fosters bigotry and racism toward other communities. Of course this is wrong. It contributes nothing to the happiness of humanity. Now more than ever we need to show our children that distinctions between "my country" and "your country," "my religion" and "your religion" are secondary considerations. Rather, we must insist on the observation that my right to happiness carries no more weight than others' right. This is not to say that I believe we should educate children to abandon or ignore the culture and historical tradition they were born into. On the contrary, it is very important they be grounded in these. It is good for children to learn to love their country, their religion, their culture, and so on. But the danger comes when this develops into narrow-minded nationalism, ethnocentricity, and religious bigotry. The example of Mahatma Gandhi is pertinent here. Even though he had a very high level of Western education, he never forgot or became estranged from the rich heritage of his Indian culture.

If education constitutes one of our most powerful weapons in our quest to bring about a better, more peaceful world, the mass media is another. As every political figure knows, they are no longer the only ones with authority in society. In addition to that of newspapers and books, radio, film, and television together have an influence over individuals unimagined a hundred years ago. This power confers great a responsibility on all who work in the media. But it also confers great responsibility on each of us who, as individuals, listen and read and watch. We, too, have a role to play. We are not powerless before the media. The control switch is in our own hand, after all.

This does not mean that I advocate bland reporting or entertainment without excitement. On the contrary, so far as investigative journalism is concerned, I respect and appreciate the media's interference. Not all public servants are honest in discharging their duties. It is appropriate, therefore, to have journalists, their noses as long as an elephant's trunk, snooping around and exposing wrongdoing where they find it. We need to know when this or that renowned individual hides a very different aspect behind a pleasant exterior. There should be no discrepancy between external appearances and the individual's inner life. It is the same person, after all. Such discrepancies suggest them to be untrustworthy. At the same time, it is vital that the investigator does not act out of improper motives. Without impartiality and without due respect for the other's rights, the investigation itself becomes tainted.

With regard to the question of the media's emphasis on sex and violence, there are many factors to consider. In the first instance, it is clear that much of the viewing public enjoys the sensations provoked by this sort of material. Secondly, I very much doubt that those producing material containing a lot of explicit sex and violence intend harm by it. Their motives are surely just commercial. As to whether this is positive or negative in itself is to my mind less important than the question of whether it can have an ethically wholesome effect. If the result of seeing a film in which there is a lot of violence is that the viewer's compassion is aroused, then perhaps that depiction of violence would be justified. But if the accumulation of violent images leads to indifference, then I think it is not. Indeed, such a hardening of heart is potentially dangerous. It leads all too easily to lack of empathy.

When the media focuses too closely on the negative aspects of human nature, there is a danger that we become persuaded that violence and aggression are its principal characteristics. This is a mistake, I believe. The fact that violence is newsworthy suggests the very opposite. Good news is not remarked on precisely because there is so much of it. Consider that at any given moment there must be hundreds of millions of acts of kindness taking place around the world. Although there will undoubtedly be many acts of violence in progress at the same time, their number is surely very much less. If therefore, the media is to be ethically responsible, it needs to reflect this simple fact.

Clearly it is necessary to regulate the media. The fact that we prevent our children from watching certain things indicates that we already discriminate between what is and is not appropriate according to different circumstances. But whether legislation is the right way to go about this is hard to judge. As in all matters of ethics, discipline is only really effective when it comes from within. Perhaps the best way to ensure that the output various media provides is healthy lies in the way we educate our children. If we bring them up to be aware of their responsibilities, they will be more disciplined when they become involved in the media.

Although it is perhaps too much to hope that the media will actually promote the ideals and principles of compassion, at least we should be able to expect that those involved will take care when there is the potential for negative impact. At least there should be no room for the incitement of negative acts such as racist violence. But beyond this, I don't know. Perhaps we might be able to find a way to connect more directly those who create stories for news and entertainment with the viewer, the reader, and the listener?

The Natural World

If there is one area in which both education and the media have a special responsibility, it is, I believe, our natural environment. Again, this responsibility has less to do with questions of right or wrong than with the question of survival. The natural world is our home. It is not necessarily sacred or holy, it is simply where we live. It is therefore in our interest to look after it. This is common sense. But only recently have the size of our population and the power of science and technology grown to the point that they can have a direct impact on nature. To put it another way, until now, Mother Earth has been able to tolerate our sloppy house habits. The stage has been reached where she can no longer accept our behavior in silence. The problems caused by environmental degradation can be seen as her response to our irresponsible behavior. She is warning us that there are limits even to her tolerance.

Nowhere are the consequences of our failure to exercise discipline in the way we relate to our environment more apparent than in the case of present-day Tibet. It is no exaggeration to say that the Tibet I grew up in was a wildlife paradise. Every traveler who visited Tibet before the middle of the twentieth century remarked on this. Animals were rarely hunted, except in the remotest areas where crops could not be grown. Indeed, it was customary for government officials annually to issue a proclamation protecting wildlife: "Nobody," it read, "however humble or noble, shall harm or do violence to the creatures of the waters or the wild." The only exceptions to this were rats and wolves.

As a young man, I recall seeing great numbers of different species whenever I traveled outside Lhasa. My chief memory of the three-month journey across Tibet from my birthplace at Takster in the east to Lhasa, where I was formally proclaimed Dalai Lama as a four-year-old boy, is of the wildlife we encountered along the way. Immense herds of *kiang* (wild asses) and *drong* (wild yak) freely roamed the great plains. Occasionally we would catch sight of shimmering herds of *gowa*, the shy Tibetan gazelle, of *wa*, the white-lipped deer, or of *tso*, our majestic antelope. I remember, too, my fascination for the little *chibi*, or pika, which would congregate on grassy areas. They were so friendly. I loved to watch the birds, the dignified *gho* (the bearded eagle) soaring high above monasteries perched up in the mountains, the flocks of geese (*nangbar*), and occasionally, at night, to hear the call of the *wookpa* (the long-eared owl).

Even in Lhasa, one did not feel in any way cut off from the natural world. In my rooms at the top of the Potala, the winter palace of the Dalai Lamas, I spent countless hours as a child studying the behavior of the red-beaked *khyungkar* which nested in the crevices of its walls. And behind the Norbulingka, the summer palace, I often saw pairs of *trung trung* (Japanese black-necked crane), birds which for me are the epitome of elegance and grace, that lived in the marshlands there. And all this is not to mention the crowning glory of Tibetan fauna: the bears and mountain foxes, the *chanku* (wolves), and *sazik* (the beautiful snow leopard), and the *sik* (lynx) which struck terror into the hearts of the nomad farmer or the gentle-faced giant panda, (*thom tra*), which is native to the border area between Tibet and China.

Sadly, this profusion of wildlife is no longer to be found. Partly due to hunting but primarily due to loss of habitat, what remains half a century after Tibet was occupied is only a fraction of what there was. Without exception, every Tibetan I have spoken with who has been back to visit Tibet after thirty to forty years has reported on a striking absence of wildlife. Whereas before wild animals would often come close to the house, today they are hardly anywhere to be seen.

Equally troubling is the devastation of Tibet's forests. In the past, the hills were all thickly wooded; today, those who have been back report that they are clean-shaven like a monk's head. The government in Beijing has admitted that the tragic flooding of western China, and further afield, is in part due to this. And yet I hear continuous reports of round-the-clock convoys of trucks carrying logs east out of Tibet. This is especially tragic given the country's mountainous terrain and harsh climate. It means that replanting requires sustained care and attention. Unfortunately, there is little evidence of this.

None of this is to say that, historically, we Tibetans were deliberately "conservationist." We were not. The idea of something called "pollution" simply never occurred to us. There is no denying we were rather spoiled in this respect. A small population inhabited a very large area with clean, dry air and an abundance of pure mountain water. This innocent attitude toward cleanliness meant that when we Tibetans went into exile, we were astonished to discover, for example, the existence of streams whose water is not drinkable. Like an only child, no matter what we did, Mother Earth tolerated our behavior. The result was that we had no proper understanding of cleanliness and hygiene. People would spit or blow their nose in the street without giving it a second thought. Indeed, saying this, I recall one elderly Khampa, a former bodyguard who used to come each day to circumambulate my residence in Dharamsala (a popular devotion). Unfortunately, he suffered greatly from bronchitis. This was exacerbated by the incense he carried. At each corner, therefore, he would pause to cough and expectorate so ferociously that I sometimes wondered whether he had come to pray or just to spit!

Over the years since our first arriving in exile, I have taken a close interest in environmental issues. The Tibetan government in exile has paid particular attention to introducing our children to their responsibilities as residents of this fragile planet. And I never hesitate to speak out on the subject whenever I am given the opportunity. In particular, I always stress the need to consider how our actions, in affecting the environment, are likely to affect others. I admit that this is very often difficult to judge. We cannot say for sure what the ultimate effects of, for example, deforestation might be on the soil and the local rainfall, let alone what the implications are for the planet's weather systems. The only clear thing is that we humans are the only species with the power to destroy the earth as we know it. The birds have no such power, nor do the insects, nor does any mammal. Yet if we have the capacity to destroy the earth, so, too, do we have the capacity to protect it.

What is essential is that we find methods of manufacture that do not destroy nature. We need to find ways of cutting down on our use of wood and other limited natural resources. I am no expert in this field, and I cannot suggest how this might be done. I know only that it is possible, given the necessary determination. For example, I recall hearing on a visit to Stockholm some years ago that, for the first time in many years, fish were returning to the river that runs through the city. Until recently, there were none due to industrial pollution. Yet this improvement was by no means the result of all the local factories closing down. Likewise, on a visit to Germany, I was shown an industrial development designed to produce no pollution. So, clearly, solutions do exist to limit damage to the natural world without bringing industry to a halt.

This does not mean that I believe we can rely on technology to overcome all our problems. Nor do I believe we can afford to continue destructive practices in anticipation of technical fixes being developed. Besides, the environment does not need fixing. It is our behavior in relation to it that needs to change. I question whether, in the case of such a massive looming disaster as that caused by the greenhouse effect, a "fix" could ever exist, even in theory. And supposing it could, we have to ask whether it would ever be feasible to apply it on the scale that would be required. What of the expense and what of the cost in terms of our natural resources? I suspect that these would be prohibitively high. There is also the fact that in many other fields—such as in the humanitarian relief of hunger—there are already insufficient funds to cover the work that could be undertaken. Therefore, even if one were to argue that the necessary funds could be raised, morally speaking this would be almost impossible to justify given such deficiencies. It would not be right to deploy huge sums simply in order to enable the industrialized nations to continue their harmful practices while people in other places cannot even feed themselves.

All this points to the need to recognize the universal dimension of our actions and, based on this, to exercise restraint. The necessity of this is forcefully demonstrated when we consider the propagation of our species. Although from the point of view of all the major religions, the more humans the better, and although it may be true that some of the latest studies suggest a population implosion a century from now, still I believe we cannot ignore this issue. As a monk, it is perhaps inappropriate for me to comment on these matters. But I believe that family planning is important. Of course, I do not mean to suggest we should not have children. Human life is a precious resource, and married couples should have children unless there are compelling reasons not to. The idea of not having children just because we want to enjoy a full life without responsibility is, I think, quite mistaken. At the same time, couples do have a duty to consider the impact our numbers have on the natural environment. This is especially true given modern technology.

Fortunately, more and more people recognize the importance of ethical discipline as a means of ensuring a healthy place to live. For this reason I am optimistic that disaster can be averted. Until comparatively recently, few people gave much thought to the effects of human activity on our planet. Yet today there are even political parties whose main concern it is. Moreover, the fact that the air we breathe, the water we drink, the forests and oceans which sustain millions of different life forms, and the climatic patterns which govern our weather systems all transcend national boundaries is a source of hope. It means that no country, no matter either how rich and powerful or how poor and weak it may be, can afford not to take action in respect to this issue.

So far as the individual is concerned, the problems resulting from our neglect of our natural environment are a powerful reminder that we all have a contribution to make. And while one person's actions may not have a significant impact, the combined effect of millions of individuals' actions certainly does. This means that it is time for all those living in the industrially developed nations to give serious thought to changing their lifestyle. Again, this is not so much a question of ethics. The fact that the population of the rest of the world has an equal right to improve their standard of living is in some ways more important than the affluent being able to continue their lifestyle. If this is to be fulfilled without causing irredeemable violence to the natural world—with all the negative consequences for happiness that this would entail—the richer countries must set an example. The cost to the planet, and thus the cost to humanity, of ever-increasing standards of living is simply too great.

Politics and Economics

We all dream of a kinder, happier world. But if we wish to make it a reality, we have to ensure that compassion inspires all our actions. This is especially true with regard to our political and economic policies. Given that probably half the world's population lacks the basic necessities of adequate food, shelter, medical care, and education, I believe we need to question whether we are really pursuing the wisest course in this regard. I think not. If it seemed likely that after another fifty years of carrying on as we are, we could definitely eradicate poverty, perhaps our present inequity of wealth distribution could be justified. Yet, on the contrary, if present trends continue, it is certain that the poor will get poorer. Our basic sense of fairness and justice alone suggests that we should not be content to let this happen.

Of course, I don't know much about economics. But I find it hard to avoid the conclusion that the wealth of the rich is maintained through neglect of the poor, especially by means of international debt. Saying this, I do not mean to suggest that the undeveloped countries have no share of responsibility for their problems. Nor can we put all social and economic ills down to politicians and public officials. I do not deny that even in the world's most established democracies it is quite usual to hear politicians making unrealistic promises and boasting about what they are going to do when elected. But these people do not drop out of the sky. So if it is true that a given country's politicians are corrupt, we tend to find that the society is itself lacking in morality and that the individuals who make up the population do not lead ethical lives. In such cases, it is not entirely fair for the electorate to criticize its politicians. On the other hand, when people possess healthy values, and where they practice ethical discipline in their own lives out of concern for others, the public officials produced by that society will quite naturally respect those same values. Each of us, therefore, has a role to play in creating a society in which respect and care for others, based on empathy, are given top priority.

So far as the application of economic policy is concerned, the same considerations apply here as to every human activity. A sense of universal responsibility is crucial. I must admit, however, that I find it a bit difficult to make practical suggestions about the application of spiritual values in the field of commerce. This is because competition has such an important role to play. For this reason, the relationship between empathy and profit is necessarily a fragile one. Still, I do not see why it should not be possible to have constructive competition. The key factor is the motivation of those engaged in it. When the intention is to exploit or destroy others, then clearly the outcome will not be positive. But when competition is conducted with a spirit of generosity and good intention, the outcome, although it must entail a degree of suffering for those who lose, will at least not be too harmful.

Again it may be objected that the reality of commerce is such that we cannot realistically expect businesses to put people before profits. But here we must remember that those who run the world's industries and businesses are human beings too. Even the most hardened would surely admit that it is not right to seek profits regardless of consequences. If it were, dealing in drugs would not be wrong. So again, what is required is that each of us develops our compassionate nature. The more we do so, the more commercial enterprise will come to reflect basic human values.

Conversely, if we ourselves neglect those values, it is inevitable that commerce will neglect them too. This is not just idealism. History shows that many of the positive developments in human society have occurred as the result of compassion. If we look at the evolution of human society, we see the necessity of having vision in order to bring about positive change. Ideals are the engine of progress. To ignore this and say merely that we need to be "realistic" in politics is severely mistaken. Consider, for example, the abolition of the slave trade.

Our problems of economic disparity pose a very serious challenge to the whole human family. Nevertheless, as we enter the new millennium, I believe there are a good number of reasons for optimism. During the early and middle years of the twentieth century, there was a general perception that political and economic power was of more consequence than truth. But I believe that this is changing. Even the wealthiest and most powerful nations understand that there is no point in neglecting basic human values. The notion that there is room for ethics in international relations is also gaining ground. Irrespective of whether it is translated into meaningful action, at least words like "reconciliation," "non-violence," and "compassion" are becoming stock phrases among politicians. This is a useful development. Then, according to my own experience, I note that when I travel abroad I am often asked to speak about peace and compassion to quite large audiences—often in excess of a thousand. I doubt very much whether these topics would have attracted such numbers forty or fifty years ago. Developments such as these indicate that collectively we humans are giving more weight to fundamental values such as justice and truth.

I also take comfort in the fact that the more the world economy evolves, the more explicitly interdependent it becomes. As a result, every nation is to a greater or lesser extent dependent on every other nation. The modern economy, like the environment, knows no boundaries. Even those countries openly hostile to one another must cooperate in their use of the world's resources. Often, for example, they will be dependent on the same rivers. And the more interdependent our economic relationships, the more interdependent must our political relationships become. Thus we have witnessed the growth of the European Union from a small caucus of trading partners into something approaching a confederation of states with a membership now well into the double figures. We see similar, though presently less well-developed, groupings throughout the world: the Association of South East Asian Nations, the Organization for African Unity, the Organization of Petroleum Exporting Countries, to name but three. Each of these testifies to the human impulse to join together for the common good and reflects the continuing evolution of human society. What began with relatively small tribal units has progressed through the foundation of city-states to nationhood and now to alliances comprising hundreds of millions of people which increasingly transcend geographical, cultural, and ethnic divisions. This is a trend which I believe will and must continue.

We cannot deny, however, that parallel to the proliferation of these political and economic alliances there is also a clear urge toward greater consolidation along the lines of ethnicity, language, religion, and culture—often in the context of violence following loosening of the bonds of nation statehood. What are we to make of this seeming paradox—the trend toward transnational cooperative groupings, on the one hand, and the impulse toward localization on the other? In fact, there need not necessarily be a contradiction between the two. We can still imagine regional communities united in trade, social policy, and security arrangements yet consisting of a multiplicity of autonomous ethnic, cultural, religious, and other groupings. There could be a legal system protecting basic human rights common to the larger community which left the constituent communities free to pursue their desired way of life. At the same time, it is important that the establishment of unions comes about voluntarily and on the basis of recognition that the interests of those concerned are better served through collaboration. They must not be imposed. Indeed, the challenge of the new millennium is surely to find ways to achieve international—or better, *inter-community*—cooperation wherein human diversity is acknowledged and the rights of all are respected.

Chapter Fourteen

PEACE AND DISARMAMENT

CHAIRMAN MAO ONCE SAID THAT POLITical power comes from the barrel of a gun. Of course it is true that violence can achieve certain short-term objectives, but it cannot obtain long-lasting ends. If we look at history, we find that in time, humanity's love of peace, justice, and freedom always triumphs over cruelty and oppression. This is why I am such a fervent believer in non-violence. Violence begets violence. And violence means only one thing: suffering. Theoretically, it is possible to conceive of a situation where the only way to prevent large-scale conflict is through armed intervention at an early stage. But the problem with this argument is that it is very difficult, if not impossible, to predict the outcome of violence. Nor can we be sure of its justness at the outset. This only becomes clear when we have the benefit of hindsight. The only certainty is that where there is violence, there is always and inevitably suffering.

Some people will say that while the Dalai Lama's devotion to non-violence is praiseworthy, it is not really practical. Actually, it is far more naive to suppose that the human-created problems which lead to violence can ever be solved through conflict.

I am convinced that the main reason so many people say the path of non-violence is impractical is because engaging in it seems daunting: we become discouraged. Nevertheless, whereas formerly it was enough to wish for peace in one's own land, or even just in one's neighborhood, today we speak of world peace. This is only appropriate. The fact of human interdependence is so explicit now: the only peace it is meaningful to speak of is world peace. Observe, for example, that non-violence was the principal characteristic of the political revolutions which swept across so much of the world during the 1980s.

One of the most hopeful aspects of the modern age is the emergence of an international peace movement. If we hear less about it today than we did at the end of the Cold War, this is perhaps because its ideals have been absorbed into mainstream consciousness. But what do I mean when I speak of peace? Are there not grounds for supposing that war is a natural, if regrettable, human activity? Here we need to make a distinction between peace as a mere absence of war and peace as a state of tranquility founded on the deep sense of security that arises from mutual understanding, tolerance of others' point of view, and respect for their rights. Peace in this sense is not what we saw in Europe during the four and a half decades of Cold War, for example. That was only approximation. The very premise on which it rested was fear and suspicion and the strange psychology of mutually assured destruction (aptly abbreviated to MAD). Indeed, the "peace" which characterized the Cold War was so precarious, so fragile, that any serious misunderstanding on the part of either side could have had disastrous consequences. Looking back, especially with the knowledge we now have of the chaotic management of weapons systems in some quarters, I think it quite miraculous that we somehow escaped destruction!

Peace is not something which exists independently of us. But nor does war. It is true that certain individuals—political leaders, policymakers, army generals—do have particularly grave responsibilities in respect to peace. However, these people do not come from nowhere. They are not born and brought up in outer space. Like us, they were nourished by their mother's milk and affection. They are members of our own human family and have been nurtured within the society which we as individuals have helped create. Peace in the world thus depends on peace in the hearts of individuals. This in turn depends on us all practicing ethics by disciplining our response to negative thoughts and emotions, and developing basic spiritual qualities.

If real peace is something more profound than

a fragile equilibrium based on mutual hostility, if ultimately it depends on the resolution of internal conflict, what are we to say about war? Although paradoxically the aim of most military campaigns is peace, in reality, war is like fire in the human community, one whose fuel is living people. It also strongly resembles fire in the way it spreads. If, for example, we look at the course of the recent conflict in the former Yugoslavia, we see that what began as a relatively confined dispute grew quickly to engulf the whole region. Similarly, if we look at individual battles, we see that where commanders perceive areas of weakness, they respond by sending in reinforcements—which is exactly like throwing live people onto a bonfire. But because of habituation, we ignore this. We fail to acknowledge that the very nature of war is cold cruelty and suffering.

The unfortunate truth is that we are conditioned to regard warfare as something exciting and even glamorous: the soldiers in smart uniforms (so attractive to children) with their military bands playing alongside them. We see murder as dreadful, but there is no association of war with criminality. On the contrary, it is seen as an opportunity for people to prove their competence and courage. We speak of the heroes it produces, almost as if the greater the number killed, the more heroic the individual. And we talk about this or that weapon as a marvelous piece of technology, forgetting that when it is used it will actually maim and murder living people. Your friend, my friend, our mothers, our fathers, our sisters and brothers, you and me.

What is even worse is the fact that in modern warfare the role of those who instigate it are often far removed from the conflict on the ground. At the same time, its impact on non-combatants grows even greater. Those who suffer most in today's armed conflicts are the innocent—not only the families of those fighting but, in far greater numbers, civilians who often do not even play a direct role. Even after the war is over, there continues to be enormous suffering due to land mines and poisoning from the use of chemical weapons—not to mention the economic hardship it brings. This means that, more and more, women, children, and the elderly are among its prime victims.

The reality of modern warfare is that the whole enterprise has become almost like a computer game. The ever-increasing sophistication of weaponry has outrun the imaginative capacity of the average layperson. Their destructive capacity is so astonishing that whatever arguments there may be in favor of war, they must be vastly inferior to those against. We could almost be forgiven for feeling nostalgia for the way in which battles were fought in ancient times. At least then people fought one another face-to-face. There was no denying the suffering involved. And in those days, it was usual for rulers to lead their troops in battle. If the ruler was killed, that was usually the end of the matter. But as technology improved, the generals began to stay farther behind. Today they can be thousands of miles away in their bunkers underground. In view of this, I could see developing a "smart" bullet that could seek out those who decide on wars in the first place. That would seem to me more fair, and on these grounds I would welcome a weapon that eliminated the decision-makers while leaving the innocent unharmed.

Because of the reality of this destructive capacity, we need to admit that, whether they are intended for offensive or for defensive purposes, weapons exist solely to destroy human beings. But lest we suppose that peace is purely dependent on disarmament, we must also acknowledge that weapons cannot act by themselves. Although designed to kill, so long as they remain in storage, they can do no physical harm. Someone has to push a button to launch a missile strike, or pull a trigger to fire a bullet. No "evil" power can do this. Only humans can. Therefore, genuine world peace requires that we also begin to dismantle the military establishments that we have built. We cannot hope to enjoy peace in its fullest sense while it remains possible for a few individuals to exercise military power and impose their will on others. Nor, for that matter, can we hope to enjoy true peace as long as there are authoritarian regimes propped up by armed forces which do not hesitate to carry out injustice at their bidding. Injustice undermines truth, and without truth there can be no lasting peace. Why not? Because when we have truth on our side, there is a straightforwardness, a confidence that comes with it. Conversely, when truth is lacking, the only way we can achieve our narrow aims is through force. But when decisions come about this way, in defiance of truth, people do not feel quite right—either the victors or the vanquished. This negative feeling serves to undermine the peace which is imposed by force.

We each have a role to play in this. When, as individuals, we disarm ourselves internally— through countering our negative thoughts and emotions and cultivating positive qualities— we create the conditions for external disarmament. Indeed, genuine, lasting world peace will only be possible as a result of each of us making an effort internally. Afflictive emotion is the oxygen of conflict. It is thus essential that we remain sensitive to others and, recognizing their equal right to happiness, do nothing that could contribute to their suffering. To help us in this, it is useful to take time to reflect on how war is actually experienced by its victims. For my own part, I need only think of my visit to Hiroshima some years ago to bring to life its full horror. In the museum there, I saw a watch that had stopped at the exact moment the bomb exploded. I also saw a small packet of sewing needles, the contents of which had been fused together in its heat.

Clearly we cannot hope to achieve military disestablishment overnight. Desirable as it may be, unilateral disarmament would be exceedingly difficult to achieve. And although if we wish to see a society in which armed conflict becomes a thing of the past, our ultimate goal must be the abolition of all military apparatus, clearly it is too much to hope for the elimination of all weapons. After all, even our fists can be used as weapons. And there will always be groups of troublemakers and fanatics who will cause disturbance for others. Therefore, we must allow that, as long as there are human beings, there will have to be ways of dealing with miscreants.

What is required, therefore, is that we establish clear objectives by means of which we can disarm gradually. And we must develop the political will to do so. With respect to the practical measures required to bring about military disestablishment, we need to recognize that it can only occur within the context of a broad commitment to disarmament. It is not enough to think merely in terms of eliminating our weapons of mass destruction. We must create the conditions favorable to our objective. The most obvious way of doing this is by building on existing initiatives. Here I am thinking of the efforts over many years to exercise control over the proliferation of certain classes of weapon—and in some cases to eliminate them. During the 1970s and 1980s, we saw the SALT (Strategic Arms Limitation Treaties) talks between the Eastern and Western blocs. We have had in place for many years a nuclear non-proliferation treaty to which many countries are already committed. And despite the spread of nuclear weapons, the idea of a universal ban is still alive. Encouraging progress has also been made toward the banning of land mines. At the time of this writing, a majority of the world's governments have signed protocols renouncing their use. So while it remains true that none of these initiatives has so far fully succeeded in their aims, their very existence indicates recognition of the undesirability of these methods of destruction. They testify to humans' basic wish to live in peace. And they provide a useful start which is capable of development.

Another way in which we can move further toward our objective of global military disestablishment is by gradually dismantling our arms industry. To many, this suggestion will seem a preposterous and unfeasible idea. They will object that unless everybody agrees to do so simultaneously, this would be madness. And that, they will say, can never happen. Besides, they will add, there is the economic argument to consider. Yet if we look at the matter from the point of view of those who suffer the consequences of armed violence, it becomes very hard to deny our responsibility to overcome these objections by some means or another. Indeed, whenever I think of the arms industry and the suffering it enables, I am again reminded of my visit to the Nazi death camp at Auschwitz. As I stood looking at the ovens in which thousands of human beings just like myself were burned—many of them still alive, humans who cannot bear the heat of a single match—what struck me hardest was the realization that these devices had been built with the care and attention of talented workmen. I could almost see the engineers (all intelligent people) at their drawing boards, carefully planning the shape of the combustion chambers and calculating the size of chimneys, their height and breadth. I thought of the craftsmen who brought the design to fruition. No doubt they took pride in their work, as good craftsmen do. Then it occurred to me that this is precisely what modern-day weapons designers and manufacturers are about. They, too, are devising the means to destroy thousands if not millions of their fellow human beings. Isn't this a disturbing thought?

With this in mind, all those individuals who undertake such work would do well to consider whether they can really justify their involvement. No doubt they would suffer if they gave it up unilaterally. No doubt, too, the economies of the arms manufacturing nations would suffer if these facilities were closed down. But would this not be a price worth paying? Besides, it seems that there are many examples in the world of companies which have successfully converted from weapons to some other form of manufacture. Also, we have the example of the world's one demilitarized state which we can consider in relation to its neighbors. If the example of Costa Rica, which disarmed as long ago as 1949, is anything to go by, the benefits in terms of standard of living, of health, and often education are tremendous.

As to the argument that it would perhaps be more realistic simply to restrict arms exports to those countries which are reliable and safe, I suggest that this reflects a very short-sighted outlook. It has been demonstrated time and time again that this does not work. We are all familiar with the recent history of the Persian Gulf. During the 1970s, the Western allies armed the Shah of Iran as a counterforce to the perceived threat from Russia. Then, when the political climate changed, Iran itself was considered a threat to Western interest. So the allies began to arm Iraq against Iran. But then, when times changed yet again, these weapons were used against the West's other allies in the Gulf (Kuwait). As a result, the manufacturing countries found themselves going to war with their own client. In other words, there is no such thing as a "safe" client for arms.

I cannot deny that my aspiration toward global disarmament and military disestablishment is idealistic. At the same time, there are clear grounds for optimism. One of these is the ironic fact that so far as nuclear and other weapons of mass destruction are concerned, it is extremely hard to conceive of a situation where they could be useful. Nobody wants to risk all-out nuclear war. These weapons are also an obvious waste of money. They are expensive to produce, it is impossible to imagine using them, and there is nothing to do but stockpile them, which also costs a great deal of money. In effect, therefore, they are utterly useless and nothing but a drain on resources.

Another reason for optimism is again the steady intertwining of national economies. This is creating a climate in which notions of purely national interest and advantage are becoming less and less meaningful. As a result, the idea of war as a means to resolve conflict is starting to look decidedly old-fashioned. Where there are human beings, there will always be conflict, this is true. Disagreements are bound to surface from time to time. But given today's reality of increasingly widespread nuclear weapons proliferation, we have to find some way other than violence to resolve them. This means dialogue in the spirit of reconciliation and compromise. This is not just wishful thinking on my part. The global trend toward international political groupings, of which the European Union is perhaps the most obvious example, means that it is possible to envisage a time when maintaining purely national standing armies could one day seem both uneconomic and unnecessary. Instead of thinking only in terms of protecting individual borders, it will become logical to think in terms of regional security. In fact, this is already beginning to happen. There are, albeit as yet tentative, plans to integrate European defenses more closely; a Franco-German army brigade has been in existence for more than ten years now. It thus seems possible, at least so far as the European Community is concerned, that what began purely as a trading alliance could eventually assume responsibility for regional security. And if this is possible within Europe, there is reason to hope that other international trading groups—of which there are many—could evolve to do the same. Why not?

The emergence of such regional security groupings would, I feel, contribute enormously to the transition from our current preoccupation with nation-states to the gradual acceptance of less narrowly defined communities. They could also pave the way for a world in which there would be no standing armies at all. Such a scenario would, of course, have to evolve in stages. National armed forces would give way to regional security groupings. These could then gradually be disbanded, leaving only a globally administered police force. The main purpose of this force would be to safeguard justice, communal security, and human rights worldwide. Its specific duties would be various, however. Protecting against the appropriation of power by violent means would be one of them. As to its operation, granted there are legal issues to be tackled first. But I imagine that it would be called in either by communities which came under threat—from neighbors or from some of its own members, such as a violently extreme political faction—or it could be deployed by the international community itself when violence seemed the likely outcome of conflict, for example, of religious or ideological disputes.

Even though it is true that we remain a long way from this ideal situation, again it is not so fanciful as it may at first seem. Maybe this generation will not live to see it. But we are already accustomed to seeing United Nations troops deployed as peacekeepers. We are also beginning to see the emergence of a consensus that under certain circumstances it may be justifiable to use them in a more interventionist way.

As a means for furthering these developments we might consider the establishment of what I call Zones of Peace. Here I imagine either a part or parts of one or more country being demilitarized to create oases of stability, preferably in areas of strategic significance. These would serve as beacons of hope for the rest of the world. Admittedly, this idea is quite ambitious, but it is not without precedent. We already have one such internationally recognized demilitarized zone in Antarctica. Nor am I the only individual ever to suggest there could be more. Former Russian President Mikhail Gorbachev proposed just such status for the Sino-Russian borderlands. I myself have advanced the idea for Tibet.

Of course, it is not hard to think of areas in the world other than Tibet where neighboring communities would benefit enormously from the establishment of a demilitarized zone. Just as India and China—both of them still relatively poor countries—would save a considerable proportion of their respective annual income if Tibet were to become an internationally recognized Zone of Peace, so there are many others on each continent from which a tremendous, wasteful burden would be lifted if there were no need to maintain large numbers of troops on their borders. I have often thought, for example, that Germany is a most appropriate location for a Zone of Peace, lying as it does in the heart of Europe and taking into account the experience of the twentieth century's two world wars.

In all of this, I believe the United Nations has a critical role to play. Not that it is the only body devoted to global issues. There is also much to admire about the ideas behind the International Court at the Hague, the International Monetary Fund, the World Bank, and others such as those dedicated to upholding the Geneva conventions. But, at present, and for the conceivable future, the United Nations is the only global institution capable of both influencing and formulating policy on behalf of the international community. Of course, many people criticize it on the grounds that it is ineffective, and it is true that time and again we have seen its resolutions ignored, abandoned, and forgotten. Nevertheless, in spite of these shortcomings, I for one continue to have the highest regard not only for the principles on which it was founded but also for the great deal it has achieved since its inception in 1945. We need only ask ourselves whether or not it has helped save lives through defusing potentially disastrous situations to see that it is more than the toothless bureaucracy some people say it is. We should also consider the great work of its subsidiary organizations, such as UNICEF, United Nations High Commission for Refugees, UNESCO, and the World Health Organization. This remains true even if some of their programs and policies and those of other world organizations have been flawed and misguided.

I see the United Nations, if it could be developed to its full potential, as being the proper vehicle for carrying out the wishes of humanity as a whole. As yet it is not able to do this very effectively, but then we are only just beginning to see the emergence of a global consciousness (which has been made possible by the communications revolution). And in spite of tremendous difficulties, we have seen it in action in numerous parts of the world, even though at the moment there may only be one or two nations spearheading these initiatives. The fact that they are seeking the legitimacy conferred by a United Nations mandate suggests a felt need for justification through collective approbation. This, in turn, I believe to be indicative of a growing sense of a single, mutually dependent, human community.

One of the particular weaknesses of the United Nations as it is presently constituted is that although it provides a forum for individual governments, individual citizens cannot be heard there. It has no mechanism whereby those wishing to speak out against their own governments can be heard. To make matters worse is the fact that the veto system currently in place opens its workings to manipulation by the more powerful nations. These are profound shortcomings.

As to the problem of individuals not having a voice, here we might have to consider something more radical. Just as democracy is ensured by the three pillars of an independent judiciary, executive, and legislature, so we need to have a genuinely independent body at the international level. But perhaps the United Nations is not entirely suited to this role. I have noticed at international gatherings, such as the Earth summit in Brazil, that individuals representing their country inevitably put their nations' interests first, despite the fact that the question at issue transcends national boundaries. Conversely, when people come as individuals to international gatherings— here I am thinking of such groups as the International Physicians for the Prevention of Nuclear War group, or the initiative on the arms trade by the Nobel Peace Laureates, of which I am a member—there is much greater concern for humanity itself. Their spirit is much more genuinely international and open. This leads me to think that it could be worthwhile to establish a body whose principal task is to monitor human affairs from the perspective of ethics, an organization that might be called the World Council of the People (although no doubt a better name could be found). This would consist in a group of individuals drawn, as I imagine it, from a wide variety of backgrounds. There would be artists, bankers, environmentalists, lawyers, poets, academics, religious thinkers, and writers as well as ordinary men and women with a common reputation for integrity and dedication to fundamental ethical and human values. Because this body would not actually be invested with political power, its pronouncements would not be legally binding. But by virtue of its independence—having no link with any one nation or group of nations, and no ideology—these deliberations would represent the conscience of the world. They would thus carry moral authority.

Of course, there will be many who criticize this proposal, along with what I have said about military disestablishment, disarmament, and reform of the United Nations on the grounds that it is unrealistic, or perhaps just too simplistic. Or they will say that it is not workable in "the real world." But while people are often content to just criticize and blame others for what goes wrong, surely we should at least attempt to put forward constructive ideas. One thing is for certain. Given human beings' love of truth, justice, peace, and freedom, creating a better, more compassionate world is a genuine possibility. The potential is there. If, with the help of education and the proper use of the media, we can combine some of the initiatives suggested here with the implementation of ethical principles, we will have within our reach a climate in which disarmament and military disestablishment become totally uncontroversial. On the basis of this we will have created the conditions for lasting world peace.

Chapter Fifteen

THE ROLE OF RELIGION IN MODERN SOCIETY

IT IS A SAD FACT OF HUMAN HISTORY that religion has been a major source of conflict. Even today, individuals are killed, communities destroyed, and societies destabilized as a result of religious bigotry and hatred. It is no wonder that many question the place of religion in human society. Yet when we think carefully, we find that conflict in the name of religion arises from two principal sources. There is that which arises simply as a result of religious diversity—the doctrinal, cultural, and practical differences between one religion and another. Then there is the conflict that arises in the context of political, economic, and other factors, mainly at the institutional level. Interreligious harmony is the key to overcoming conflict of the first sort. In the case of the second, some other solution must be found. Secularization and in particular the separation of the religious hierarchy from the institutions of the state may go some way to reducing such institutional problems. Our concern in this chapter is with interreligious harmony, however.

This is an important aspect of what I have called universal responsibility. But before examining the matter in detail, it is perhaps worth considering the question of whether religion is really relevant in the modern world. Many people argue that it is not. Now I have observed that religious belief is not a precondition either of ethical conduct or of happiness itself. I have also suggested that whether a person practices religion or not, the spiritual qualities of love and compassion, patience, tolerance, forgiveness, humility, and so on are indispensable. At the same time, I should make it clear that I believe that these are most easily and effectively developed within the context of religious practice. I also believe that when an individual sincerely practices religion, that individual will benefit enormously. People who have developed a firm faith, grounded in understanding and rooted in daily practice, are in general much better at coping with adversity than those who have not. I am convinced, therefore, that religion has enormous potential to benefit humanity. Properly employed, it is an extremely effective instrument for establishing human happiness. In particular, it can play a leading role in encouraging people to develop a sense of responsibility toward others and of the need to be ethically disciplined.

On these grounds, therefore, I believe that religion is still relevant today. But consider this too: some years ago, the body of a Stone Age man was recovered from the ice of the European Alps. Despite being more than five thousand years old, it was perfectly preserved. Even its clothes were largely intact. I remember thinking at the time that were it possible to bring this individual back to life for a day, we would find that we have much in common with him. No doubt we would find that he too was concerned for his family and loved ones, for his health and so on. Differences of culture and expression notwithstanding, we would still be able to identify with one another on the level of feeling. And there could be no reason to suppose any less concern with finding happiness and avoiding suffering on his part than on ours. If religion, with its emphasis on overcoming suffering through the practice of ethical discipline and cultivation of love and compassion, can be conceived of as relevant in his time, it is hard to see why it should not be equally so today. Granted that in the past the value of religion may have been more obvious in that human suffering was more explicit due to the lack of modern facilities. But because we humans still suffer, albeit today this is experienced more internally as mental and emotional affliction, and because religion in addition to its salvific truth claims is concerned to help us overcome suffering, surely it must still be relevant.

How then might we bring about the harmony

that is necessary to overcome interreligious conflict? As in the case of individuals engaged in the discipline of restraining their response to negative thoughts and emotions and cultivating spiritual qualities, the key lies in developing understanding. We must first identify the factors that obstruct it. Then we must find ways to overcome them.

Perhaps the most significant obstruction to interreligious harmony is lack of appreciation of the value of others' faith traditions. Until comparatively recently, communication between different cultures, even different communities, was slow or nonexistent. For this reason, sympathy for other faith traditions was not necessarily very important—except of course where members of different religions lived side by side. But this attitude is no longer viable. In today's increasingly complex and interdependent world, we are compelled to acknowledge the existence of other cultures, different ethnic groups, and, of course, other religious faiths. Whether we like it or not, most of us now experience this diversity on a daily basis.

I believe that the best way to overcome ignorance and bring about understanding is through dialogue with members of other faith traditions. This I see occurring in a number of different ways. Discussions among scholars in which the convergence and perhaps more importantly the divergence between different faith traditions are explored and appreciated are very valuable. On another level, it is helpful when there are encounters between ordinary but practicing followers of different religions in which each shares their experiences. This is perhaps the most effective way of appreciating others' teachings. In my own case, for example, my meetings with the late Thomas Merton, a Catholic monk of the Cistercian order, were deeply inspiring. They helped me develop a profound admiration for the teachings of Christianity. I also feel that occasional meetings between religious leaders joining together to pray for a common cause are extremely useful. The gathering at Assisi in Italy in 1986, when representatives of the world's major religions gathered to pray for peace, was, I believe, tremendously beneficial to many religious believers insofar as it symbolized the solidarity and a commitment to peace of all those taking part.

Finally, I feel that the practice of members of different faith traditions going on joint pilgrimages together can be very helpful. It was in this spirit that in 1993 I went to Lourdes, and then to Jerusalem—a site holy to three of the world's great religions. I have also paid visits to various Hindu, Islamic, Jain, and Sikh shrines both in India and abroad. More recently, following a seminar devoted to discussing and practicing meditation in the Christian and Buddhist traditions, I joined an historic pilgrimage of practitioners of both traditions in a program of prayers, meditation, and dialogue under the Bodhi tree at Bodh Gaya in India. This is one of Buddhism's most important shrines.

When exchanges like these occur, followers of one tradition will find that, just as in the case of their own, the teachings of others faiths are a source both of spiritual inspiration and of ethical guidance to their followers. It will also become clear that irrespective of doctrinal and other differences, all the major world religions are concerned with helping individuals to become good human beings. All emphasize love and compassion, patience, tolerance, forgiveness, humility, and so on, and all are capable of helping individuals to develop these. Moreover, the example given by the founders of each major religion clearly demonstrates a concern for helping others find happiness through developing these qualities. So far as their own lives were concerned, each conducted themselves with great simplicity. Ethical discipline and love for all others was the hallmark of their lives. They did not live luxuriously like emperors and kings. Instead, they voluntarily accepted suffering— without consideration of the hardships involved—in order to benefit humanity as a whole. In their teachings, all placed special emphasis on developing love and compassion and renouncing selfish desires. And each of them called on us to transform our hearts and minds. Indeed, whether we have faith or not, all are worthy of our profound admiration.

At the same time as engaging in dialogue with followers of other religions, we must, of course, implement in our daily life the teachings of our own religion. Once we have experienced the benefit of love and compassion, and of ethical discipline, we will easily recognize the value of other's teachings. But for this, it is essential to realize that religious practice entails a lot more than merely saying, "I believe" or, as in Buddhism, "I take refuge." There is also more to it than just visiting temples, or shrines, or churches. And taking religious teachings is of little benefit if they do not enter the heart but remain at the level of intellect alone. Simply relying on faith without understanding and without implementation is of limited value. I often tell Tibetans that carrying a *mala* (something like a rosary) does not make a person a genuine religious practitioner. The efforts we make sincerely to transform ourselves spiritually are what make us genuine religious practitioners.

We come to see the overriding importance of genuine practice when we recognize that, along with ignorance, individuals' unhealthy relationships with their beliefs is the other major factor in religious disharmony. Far from applying the teachings of their religion in our personal lives, we have a tendency to use them to reinforce our self-centered attitudes. We relate to our religion as something we own or as a label that separates us from others. Surely this is misguided? Instead of using the nectar of religion to purify the poisonous elements of our hearts and minds, there is a danger when we think like this of using these negative elements to poison the nectar of religion.

Yet we must acknowledge that this reflects another problem, one which is implicit in all religions. I refer to the claims each has of being the one "true" religion. How are we to resolve this difficulty? It is true that from the point of view of the individual practitioner, it is essential to have a single-pointed commitment to one's own faith. It is also true that this depends on the deep conviction that one's own path is the sole mediator of truth. But at the same time, we have to find some means of reconciling this belief with the reality of a multiplicity of similar claims. In practical terms, this involves individual practitioners finding a way at least to accept the validity of the teachings of other religions while maintaining a whole-hearted commitment to their own. As far as the validity of the metaphysical truth claims of a given religion is concerned, that is of course the internal business of that particular tradition.

In my own case, I am convinced that Buddhism provides me with the most effective framework within which to situate my efforts to develop spiritually through cultivating love and compassion. At the same time, I must acknowledge that while Buddhism represents the best path for me—that is, it suits my character, my temperament, my inclinations, and my cultural background—the same will be true of Christianity for Christians. For them, Christianity is the best way. On the basis of my conviction, I cannot, therefore, say that Buddhism is best for everyone.

I often think of religion in terms of medicine for the human spirit. Independent of its usage and suitability to a particular individual in a particular condition, we really cannot judge a medicine's efficacy. We are not justified in saying this medicine is very good because of such and such ingredients. If you take the patient and the medicine's effect on that person out of the equation, it hardly makes sense. What is relevant is to say that in the case of this particular patient with his or her particular illness, this medicine is the most effective. Similarly with different religious traditions, we can say that this one is most effective for this particular individual. But it is unhelpful to try to argue on the basis of philosophy or metaphysics that one religion is better than another. The important thing is surely its effectiveness in individual cases.

My way to resolve the seeming contradiction between each religion's claim to "one truth and one religion" and the reality of the multiplicity of faiths is thus to understand that in the case of a single individual, there can indeed be only one truth, one religion. However, from the perspective of human society at large, we must accept the concept of "many truths, many religions." To continue with our medical analogy, in the case of one particular patient, the suitable medicine is in fact the only medicine. But clearly that does not mean that there may not be other medicines suitable to other patients.

To my way of thinking, the diversity that

exists among the various religious traditions is enormously enriching. There is thus no need to try to find ways of saying that ultimately all religions are the same. They are similar in that they all emphasize the indispensability of love and compassion in the context of ethical discipline. But to say this is not to say that they are all essentially one. The contradictory understanding of creation and beginninglessness articulated by Buddhism, Christianity, and Hinduism, for example, means that in the end we have to part company when it comes to metaphysical claims, in spite of the many practical similarities that undoubtedly exist. These contradictions may not be very important in the beginning stages of religious practice. But as we advance along the path of one tradition or another, we are compelled at some point to acknowledge fundamental differences. For example, the concept of rebirth in Buddhism and various other ancient Indian traditions may turn out to be incompatible with the Christian idea of salvation. This need not be a cause for dismay, however. Even within Buddhism itself, in the realm of metaphysics there are diametrically opposing views. At the very least, such diversity means that we have different frameworks within which to locate ethical discipline and the development of spiritual values. That is why I do not advocate a "super" or a new "world" religion. It would mean that we would lose the unique characteristics of the different faith traditions.

Some people, it is true, hold that the Buddhist concept of *shunyata,* or emptiness, is ultimately the same as certain approaches to understanding the concept of God. Nevertheless, there remain difficulties with this. The first is that while of course we can interpret these concepts, to what extent can we be faithful to the original teachings if we do so? There are compelling similarities between the Mahayana Buddhist concept of *dharmakaya, sambogakaya,* and *nirmanakaya* and the Christian trinity of God as Father, Son, and Holy Spirit. But to say, on the basis of this, that Buddhism and Christianity are ultimately the same is to go a bit far, I think! As an old Tibetan saying goes, we must beware of trying to put a yak's head on a sheep's body—or vice versa.

What is required instead is that we develop a genuine sense of religious pluralism in spite of the different claims of different faith traditions. This is especially true if we are serious in our respect for human rights as a universal principle. In this regard, I find the concept of a world parliament of religions very appealing. To begin with, the word "parliament" conveys a sense of democracy, while the plural "religions" underlines the importance of the principle of a multiplicity of faith traditions. The truly pluralist perspective on religion which the idea of such a parliament suggests could, I believe be, of great help. It would avoid the extremes of religious bigotry on the one hand, and the urge toward unnecessary syncretism on the other.

Connected with this issue of interreligious harmony, I should perhaps say something about religious conversion. This is a question which must be taken extremely seriously. It is essential to realize that the mere fact of conversion alone will not make an individual a better person—that is to say, a more disciplined, a more compassionate, a more warm-hearted person. Much more helpful, therefore, is for the individual to concentrate on transforming themselves spiritually through the practice of restraint, virtue, and compassion. To the extent that the insights or practices of other religions are useful or relevant to our own faith, it is valuable to learn from others. In some cases, it may even be helpful to adopt certain of them. Yet when this is done wisely, we can remain firmly committed to our own faith. This way is best because it carries with it no danger of confusion, especially with respect to the different ways of life that tend to go with different faith traditions.

Given the diversity to be found among individual human beings, it is of course bound to be the case that out of many millions of practitioners of a particular religion, a handful will find that another religion's approach to ethics and spiritual development is more satisfactory. For some, the concept of rebirth and karma will seem highly effective in inspiring the aspiration to develop love and compassion within the context of responsibility. For others, the concept of a transcendent, loving creator will come to seem more so. In such circumstances, it is crucial for those individuals to question themselves again and again. They must ask, "Am I attracted to this other religion for the right reasons? Is it merely the cultural and ritual aspects that are appealing? Or is it the essential teachings? Do I suppose that if I convert to this new religion it will be less demanding than my present one?" I say this because it has often struck me that when people do convert to a religion outside their own heritage, quite often they adopt certain superficial aspects of the culture to which their new faith belongs. But their practice may not go very much deeper than that.

In the case of a person who decides after a process of long and mature reflection to adopt a different religion, it is very important that they remember the positive contribution to humanity of each religious tradition. The danger is that the individual may, in seeking to justify their decision to others, criticize their previous faith. It is essential to avoid this. Just because that tradition is no long effective in the case of one individual does not mean it is no longer of benefit to humanity. On the contrary, we can be certain that it has been an inspiration to millions of people in the past, that it inspires millions today, and that it will inspire millions in the path of love and compassion in the future.

The important point to keep in mind is that ultimately the whole purpose of religion is to facilitate love and compassion, patience, tolerance, humility, forgiveness, and so on. If we neglect these, changing our religion will be of no help. In the same way, even if we are fervent believers in our own faith, it will avail us nothing if we neglect to implement these qualities in our daily lives. Such a believer is no better off than a patient with some fatal illness who merely reads a medical treatise but fails to undertake the treatment prescribed.

Moreover, if we who are practitioners of religion are not compassionate and disciplined, how can we expect it of others? If we can establish genuine harmony derived from mutual respect and understanding, religion has enormous potential to speak with authority on such vital moral questions as peace and disarmament, social and political justice, the natural environment, and many other matters affecting all humanity. But until we put our own spiritual teachings into practice, we will never be taken seriously. And this means, among other things, setting a good example through developing good relations with other faith traditions.

Chapter Sixteen

AN APPEAL

THAT WE HAVE REACHED THE LAST FEW pages of this book reminds us of the impermanence of our lives. How quickly they pass and how soon we will arrive at our final day. Within less than fifty years, I, Tenzin Gyatso, the Buddhist monk, will be no more than a memory. Indeed, it is doubtful whether a single person reading these words will be alive a century from now. Time passes unhindered. When we make mistakes, we cannot turn the clock back and try again. All we can do is use the present well. Therefore, if when our final day comes we are able to look back and see that we have lived full, productive, and meaningful lives, that will at least be of some comfort. If we cannot, we may be very sad. But which of these we experience is up to us.

The best way to ensure that when we approach death we do so without remorse is to ensure that in the present moment we conduct ourselves responsibly and with compassion for others. Actually, this is in our own interest, and not just because it will benefit us in the future. As we have seen, compassion is one of the principal things that make our lives meaningful. It is the source of all lasting happiness and joy. And it is the foundation of a good heart, the heart of one who acts out of a desire to help others. Through kindness, through affection, through honesty, through truth and justice toward all others we ensure our own benefit. This is not a matter for complicated theorizing. It is a matter of common sense. There is no denying that consideration of others is worthwhile. There is no denying that our happiness is inextricably bound up with the happiness of others. There is no denying that if society suffers, we ourselves suffer. Nor is there any denying that the more our hearts and minds are afflicted with ill-will, the more miserable we become. Thus we can reject everything else: religion, ideology, all received wisdom. But we cannot escape the necessity of love and compassion.

This, then, is my true religion, my simple faith. In this sense, there is no need for temple or church, for mosque or synagogue, no need for complicated philosophy, doctrine, or dogma. Our own heart, our own mind, is the temple. The doctrine is compassion. Love for others and respect for their rights and dignity, no matter who or what they are: ultimately these are all we need. So long as we practice these in our daily lives, then no matter if we are learned or unlearned, whether we believe in Buddha or God, or follow some other religion or none at all, as long as we have compassion for others and conduct ourselves with restraint out of a sense of responsibility, there is no doubt we will be happy.

Why, then, if it is so simple to be happy, do we find it so hard? Unfortunately, though most of us think of ourselves as compassionate, we tend to ignore these common-sense truths. We neglect to confront our negative thoughts and emotions. Unlike the farmer who follows the seasons and does not hesitate to cultivate the land when the moment comes, we waste so much of our time in meaningless activity. We feel deep regret over trivial matters like losing money while keeping from doing what is genuinely important without the slightest feeling of remorse. Instead of rejoicing in the opportunity we have to contribute to others' well-being, we merely take our pleasures where we can. We shrink from considering others on the grounds that we are too busy. We run right and left, making calculations and telephone calls and thinking that this would be better than that. We do one thing but worry that if something else comes along we had better do another. But in this, we engage only the coarsest and most elementary levels of the human spirit. Moreover, by being inattentive to the needs of others, inevitably we end up harming them. We think ourselves very clever, but how do we use our abilities? All too often we use them to deceive our neighbors, to take advantage of them and better ourselves at their expense. And when things do not work out, full of self-righteousness, we blame them for our difficulties.

Yet lasting satisfaction cannot be derived from the acquisition of objects. No matter how many friends we acquire, they cannot make us happy. And indulgence in sensual pleasure is nothing but a gateway to suffering. It is like honey smeared along the cutting edge of a sword. Of course, that is not to say that we should despise our bodies. On the contrary, we cannot be of help to others without a body. But we need to avoid the extremes which can lead to harm.

In focusing on the mundane, what is essential remains hidden from us. Of course, if we could be truly happy doing so, then it would be entirely reasonable to live like this. Yet we cannot. At best, we get through life without too much trouble. But then when problems assail us, as they must, we are unprepared. We find that we cannot cope. We are left despairing and unhappy.

Therefore, with my two hands joined, I appeal to you the reader to ensure that you make the rest of your life as meaningful as possible. Do this by engaging in spiritual practice if you can. As I hope I have made clear, there is nothing mysterious about this. It consists in nothing more than acting out of concern for others. And provided you undertake this practice sincerely and with persistence, little by little, step by step you will gradually be able to reorder your habits and attitudes so that you think less about your own narrow concerns and more of others'. In doing so, you will find that you enjoy peace and happiness yourself.

Relinquish your envy, let go your desire to triumph over others. Instead, try to benefit them. With kindness, with courage, and confident that in doing so you are sure to meet with success, welcome others with a smile. Be straightforward. And try to be impartial. Treat everyone as if they were a close friend. I say this neither as Dalai Lama nor as someone who has special powers or ability. Of these I have none. I speak as a human being: one who, like yourself, wishes to be happy and not to suffer.

If you cannot, for whatever reason, be of help

to others, at least don't harm them. Consider yourself a tourist. Think of the world as it is seen from space, so small and insignificant yet so beautiful. Could there really be anything to be gained from harming others during our stay here? Is it not preferable, and more reasonable, to relax and enjoy ourselves quietly, just as if we were visiting a different neighborhood? Therefore, if in the midst of your enjoyment of the world you have a moment, try to help in however small a way those who are downtrodden and those who, for whatever reason, cannot or do not help themselves. Try not to turn away from those whose appearance is disturbing, from the ragged and unwell. Try never to think of them as inferior to yourself. If you can, try not even to think of yourself as better than the humblest beggar. You will look the same in your grave.

To close with, I would like to share a short prayer which gives me great inspiration in my quest to benefit others:

> *May I become at all times, both now*
> *and forever*
> *A protector for those without protection*
> *A guide for those who have lost their way*
> *A ship for those with oceans to cross*
> *A bridge for those with rivers to cross*
> *A sanctuary for those in danger*
> *A lamp for those without light*
> *A place of refuge for those who lack shelter*
> *And a servant to all in need.*